Weekends *at* Bellevue

Weekends *at* Bellevue

Julie Holland, M.D.

Bantam 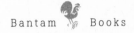 Books

Published in the United States by Bantam Books, an imprint of The Random House
Publishing Group, a division of Random House, Inc., New York.

BANTAM BOOKS and the rooster colophon are registered trademarks
of Random House, Inc.

LIBRARY OF CONGRESS CATALOGING-IN-PUBLICATION DATA

Holland, Julie
Weekends at Bellevue / Julie Holland.
p. cm.
ISBN 978-0-553-80766-0
1. Holland, Julie   2. Psychiatric emergencies—New York
(State)—New York.   3. Bellevue Hospital.   4. Emergency physicians—New
York (State)—New York—Biography.   5. Women psychiatrists—New
York (State)—New York—Biography.   I. Title.
RC480.6.H655 2009   362.2'1097471—dc22   2009021187

Printed in the United States of America on acid-free paper

www.bantamdell.com

2 4 6 8 9 7 5 3 1

First Edition

Book design by Diane Hobbing

For Wendy

Note to the Reader

There was a particularly dramatic nine-year period in my life when I was working in the psychiatric emergency room at Bellevue Hospital, surrounded by other doctors, nurses, hospital personnel—and insanity.

Though I have done my best to portray this time in writing, it is impossible to do Bellevue justice, and I knew that from the start. Everything you will read in this book actually happened, but the Bellevue experience is unique and cannot adequately be captured by any one person's interpretation. My mind's eye's version of the events will of course differ from someone else's.

Due to the sensitive nature of the circumstances, I have changed some of the identifying details to protect people's privacy, and I have changed the names of all of my colleagues and patients, except for those who have appeared in the news. Also, the chronology of some events may have been condensed, dragged out, or rearranged, but if I make a point of saying how busy it was on a given night, then I have not inflated the numbers, and if I mention what a coincidence it was that two things happened simultaneously, then they did.

The dialogue in *Weekends at Bellevue* was often transcribed virtually word for word, from notes I wrote when I got home, which I did to help exorcise the demons of the previous two days at work. When I didn't have the benefit of working from detailed notes, I tried to preserve the gist of what was said, but cannot claim to have reconstructed every conversation verbatim.

For simplicity's sake, I have tended to use "he" instead of "he or she" for third-person references that are not specific. Please forgive this; it just makes for easier reading.

I want to thank each patient, doctor, nurse, social worker, hospital police officer, New York City cop, ambulance driver, and federal agent with whom I ever came into contact during my nine years at Bellevue. If you have ended up in this book, please do not take offense. I never meant to betray your confidences, only to enlighten others with educational or entertaining stories. And we had some laughs, didn't we?

I have learned so much from my patients over the years. The purpose of this book, above all, is to share what I have learned, in the hopes that it may help people to understand some of what I feel is the "human condition" in psychiatric medicine. I am deeply grateful to all whose lives were shared with me, and who will now help in the process of educating others.

One thing needs to be explicitly clear: This is a skewed sampling of patients. Inevitably, the people whom I've chosen to write about were more colorful, dramatic, provocative, or violent than the average Bellevue patient. The vast majority of people living with psychiatric symptoms are scattered among us, *are* us, the walking wounded, and do not tend toward violence or addiction. But when I came home Monday morning and wrote down my recollections of the events of the preceding weekend, it was not to tell the tales of the garden-variety depressed or anxious patients. They, like the more seriously ill patients, deserve our tender ministrations, but I knew they wouldn't be as compelling to write or read about.

Bellevue is a great hospital that does great work, and I am proud to have been a part of this noble institution.

Weekends *at* Bellevue

Mother Nature's Son

On a warm day in early spring, two New York City cops and two EMS workers roll a gurney down the hallway, escorting a man to the entrance of Bellevue's psychiatric emergency room, where I work. Lying on the stretcher underneath a white sheet, with a head of dirty blond hair beaded and dreadlocked, he is naked, sunburned, and screaming. I walk out to greet my new patient as the drivers hand me his paperwork to sign.

"What'd you bring me?" I ask eagerly. I can see he's a live one. I love the live ones.

Over the shrieking, one of the EMS guys gives me "the bullet," the few pieces of relevant information when introducing a patient to a doctor: age, chief complaint, pertinent history. "This is Joshua Silver. Twenty-three. No significant medical history, no allergies, no meds. Also, he denies a psych history," he says archly, shooting me a look.

"And how'd he get to you guys? Who called 911?"

"NYPD called in an EDP." This is cop-talk for a psychiatric patient: emotionally disturbed person. "He'd taken off his clothes in Times Square and was parading around, barking like a dog. And growling," he adds.

This gets the patient's attention, and he interrupts the driver to clarify, "It was my way of showing them that I was not an animal. I am not a dog!"

Barking and growling to prove he is not a dog? His logic is lost on me, but at least he's stopped yelling and started communicating.

"You can talk to me," I say, turning my full attention toward him.

"See, there were some guys from Nation of Islam preaching on the corner, and they told a woman who was arguing with them that she was just a dog—God spelled backwards—to which I took offense." He then explains to me, as he did to them, that all people are art. " 'Thou art art,' I told them. 'Once you accept that all people, all objects, are art, you will live in heaven as I do.' "

"You know what, Joshua?" I ask, having decided it is time to move out of the triage area and into the locked area. "I think you and I should go talk about this inside." I want us to sit in an interview room so I can try to get some more history, and I don't feel like standing over him while he lies on a stretcher. I can already tell he's an admission and will need to be in the detainable area for patients awaiting beds upstairs.

I let EMS and NYPD know that they are free to leave, and I grab my new patient some hospital pajamas. I help him off the stretcher, wrapping his sheet around him, and walk him into the larger, locked part of the ER. As I escort him through the entrance, the door clicks definitively behind us, and I hope he doesn't notice that he is now locked in. Because he is naked, we can dispense with the contraband search, which is good. The search is often the point where people become uncooperative and agitated, ending up restrained and medicated.

Prior to entering the detainable area, a patient must remove his belt, shoelaces, rosary beads—anything that can be used to hang himself or choke a fellow patient. Inevitably, the patient will insist that he is not suicidal or dangerous, but it doesn't matter; these items are not allowed in the detainable area. Neither are cell phones, crack pipes, backpacks, knives, pens, wallets, and the list goes on. The patient has to give up just about everything along with his freedom.

Luckily, Joshua is oblivious. I show him to the bathroom where he puts on the pajamas quickly. I alternate between keeping an eye on him and setting up the interview room. There are several windowed rooms within the detainable area, each with a desk and two chairs. I put my chair closer to the door. As we settle into our talk, the first thing I notice is that although he is disheveled, he seems well-educated with an impressive vocabulary. He tells me he has written a twenty-eight-page manuscript, which he calls a prose-poem, based on his newly embraced credo that everything is art. He is hoping to reach millions of people by delivering his manifesto on the Howard Stern show on K-ROCK, a radio station in the city.

"I am a holy man," he tells me, explaining how his writing has elevated him to this level. "I feel like King Arthur in a tower of Babel." He is hyper-verbal, spewing non sequiturs. I try to keep up with him, playing follow the leader, as if we are hopping from rock to rock in a rushing stream, but he is pulling far ahead of me. Eventually, I have to tell him he's not making a lot of sense.

"Joshua, you need to slow down. I want to understand what you're saying, but it's difficult for me. I'm focusing on the illogical connections that you're making. . . ."

It sounds like "theological connections" to him, and his smile beams; he's pleased that I've grasped his religious message. I don't bother to correct him.

Being preoccupied with religion is a classic manic symptom, and mania is the better-known half of manic depression, now called bipolar disorder. In a manic state, people have less desire for sleep; they will talk more, create more, do more. Commonly, bipolar patients get hyper-religious in their newfound frenzy and sometimes end up on a street corner and then a psych ER explaining that they are Jesus or the Messiah, or that they've discovered a new religion. They've been touched by the Lord who spoke to them. They've had a vision, an epiphany, and they want to share it with the world. Their grandiosity can be charismatic and alluring. Religions and cults are formed around this kind of energy, and I'm happy to warm myself by Joshua's fire during the interview.

In March and April, our ER becomes crowded with manic patients. For many bipolars, there is a seasonality to their symptoms. Just as more people get depressed in the winter months, increased exposure to bright sunlight can elevate moods. Also, the air is heady with religious themes during spring, when Easter and Passover coincide. The resurrection is reenacted in the budding trees and sprouting flowers, miraculously coming to life where once lay a blanket of snow. We get multiple Jesuses in the ER this time of year.

Joshua's pressured speech is another sign of his mania. It rambles hither and yon, like a butterfly dancing merrily among the flowers, setting down briefly on the themes of religion and art as if they were particularly colorful blossoms. I try to join him in his wordplay, to engage him gently in the hopes of learning more about him: where he's from, where his parents are, and whether he's stopped his medication, which is a good bet. Most of the manic patients who come through our doors have gone off their meds. The mood stabilizers have significant side effects, and people are often resentful about having to use them. Also, mania usually feels better than being medicated, at least for a while. It's a bit like surfing, knowing it has to end with the inevitable wipeout, but loving the balancing act required to keep it going.

Most of our patients battle with their need for medications. When they start to feel better, they abandon their treatment plan, thinking they're cured. Even if they know they'll get sick again, they hate taking the pills so much that they stop anyway. Coming through our doors is a painful and humbling lesson in how to manage their illness.

"Joshua," I begin yet again.

"I fought the battle of Jericho."

"I've heard that about you, yes." I smile. "Are you from Jericho?" I ask earnestly.

"No, I don't think so."

"Or maybe a town near there? You took a bus to New York City from where?" I ask. "Can you tell me where your parents live? Is there anyone who might be worried about you, who doesn't know where you are?"

A town near Jericho? What the hell am I thinking? I'll tell you: I am trying to meet him where he is, to work within his delusions and focus on what's important to him, and then gently lead him out to where I am, in reality. This is one definition of psychotic—broken with reality. He lives in a dream, but his hallucinations and delusions are as real to him as the movies we star in while we sleep.

Despite my coaxing, I can't get anything useful out of him. I want to find his parents because I need to talk to someone who knows him to learn whether he's been sick like this before. And I want to let them know that he's been found. I've made dozens of phone calls to parents of the bipolar kids who end up on our doorstep. We get plenty of "first breaks" at Bellevue, the first episodes of psychosis that often herald the arrival of bipolar disorder or schizophrenia. They tend to occur in the late teens or early twenties. This is when the brain is pruning back and reorganizing connections made throughout adolescence, and also when everything is getting more challenging: starting college, joining the army, traveling. Sometimes, during these phone calls, I hear about how bright and promising their children were before they got sick. Other times, when it's not the first break, but the latest in a long series of them, the parent on the phone is terse and angry, burned-out, tired of being woken up in the middle of the night to answer the same questions from yet another psychiatrist. In many ways, that's easier for me to deal with than the heartbreak of talking to the "new" parents, giving the first diagnosis, gingerly explaining the illness and its treatment, knowing as I do that they may be in for decades of calls from ER docs.

But tonight there is no phone conversation with the Silvers. Joshua won't even acknowledge that they exist, and I have nothing to go on but his manic ramblings. He tells me he's come to New York City with three dollars in his pocket and nowhere to stay. Knowing no one in the city, he made his way from the Port Authority bus terminal to the K-ROCK radio station at five a.m. in order to spread his message. When I first started my job at Bellevue, I heard the Port Authority referred to as The Port of Atrocities, because EMS brought us such sick people from there. That name stuck with me throughout my tenure at the hospital.

Joshua continues, chronicling the events of his day. After K-ROCK turned him away, he spent the rest of the morning sleeping in Central Park. Later in the afternoon, the police in the park told him to move on, and gave him a tip: Try hanging out around Forty-Second and Broadway. Wandering around Times Square, he happened upon some teens entertaining the tourists by playing drums on overturned white plastic buckets. He danced for them, and the tourists threw him money and took his picture.

"You know how there's cops there on horses? They let me pet the horses; they seemed cool about me touching the animals, and the tourists took my picture again!" He seems impressed that he'd become a tourist attraction himself.

"Well, weren't you naked by then?" I remind him.

He admits that he must have been by this point, but then begins to digress into a tirade against photographers, who, instead of living life and immersing themselves in their surroundings, only interact superficially by documenting the scene.

"You may have a point there," I offer. I think of my boyfriend the photographer whom I confronted with exactly this accusation not so long ago.

My patient perceives me as a friend and ally because I am aligning with him, chatting agreeably rather than asking the standard annoying psychiatrist questions. There's no need for those as far as I'm concerned—he's a definite admission. The only uncertainty is whether I can get him to sign in voluntarily or will have to fill out the 9.39 paperwork for commitment.

The criterion for a 9.39 is danger to self or others, or an inability to care for self. If a patient doesn't fit this narrow definition, he needs to sign in voluntarily. A frustrating situation often develops in a family when a patient clearly needs psychiatric help but is unwilling to agree to a hospitalization. In Joshua's case, I can probably justify the danger-to-self scenario. He can't fend for himself while he's psychotic like this: He's on the street with three dollars in his pocket—that is, when he's got his pants on—eating and drinking nearly nothing.

Could severe dehydration and low blood sugar be affecting his behavior? Is he high from LSD or PCP? My money is on mania, the "working diagnosis," but it's my job to second-guess myself. If it's drug-induced, he'll come down in a day or so, but the mania won't de-escalate that rapidly. I can ask the nurses to obtain a urine sample to be tested for PCP—phencyclidine—a tranquilizer called Sernyl, once FDA-approved but now illegal. When people are high on PCP, they frequently disrobe and run amok. There is a saying among toxicologists that "naked running is PCP until proven otherwise." Since Joshua presented to the ER naked and disorganized, I figure I should at least send for the test.

If I could just talk to his parents, I'd get a sense of his history—whether he's been depressed or manic before, and what meds work best for him. Of course, he won't offer me any telephone numbers for his family, only for K-ROCK, a number he knows by heart. He still wants Howard Stern to broadcast his manifesto.

I push forward on my chosen tack: schmooze-fest. I tell him I admire his theory that people are art. I share his appreciation for the perfection of all he surveys, of the complexities and magic in the world around us. Like being high on hallucinogens, mania can provide a sense of wonder and awe at the realization of how the universe works. It's easier to access the macro, to pull back and see the big picture. Often there is a feeling that "everything is connected," a realization in common with experiences on psychedelics and with mystical religious epiphanies. There are likely neurochemical similarities between the mystical, psychedelic, and manic states.

At Bellevue, I am repeatedly shown the big picture, taught that there is more than one way to look at just about everything. When I open my ears and mind to the "ravings of a madman," I'm reminded to pay more attention, to Be Here Now. Everywhere we choose to see it, the world is full of splendor and wonderment. I'll never forget the manic teenage boy who tapped my shoulder in the detainable area, excited to explain to me that, "We're part of this huge experiment. All of us are under one microscope, being observed and studied. You know where the eyepiece of the microscope is?" he asked me, his pupils dilated with enlightenment. He pointed to the ceiling, "It's what *you* call the sun."

This is why I keep working here.

As the interview progresses, Joshua allows me to see more of his world. He tells me that he can make his dreams become real—he simply thinks of something and so makes it happen. He is convinced that he can conjure up reality out of thin air, and he spends considerable time explaining this to me. At one point in the interview he accuses me of making him crazy; the next second he considerately asks if he is making *me* crazy. He drags me deeper into our discussion as the lines between reality and fantasy blur and blend. The shifting definitions seem to include where he stops and I start. He embroiders on this theme, how there are no barriers, no boundaries between us. He explains to me how we are molecules connected, how the space between us is an illusion, not empty space but vibrating balls of energy. He touches my calf for a moment to make this point. It is rare to be touched like that by a patient; he bends down at the waist to reach the lower leg of my jeans and I wonder why he has chosen that particular part of my body to make physical contact.

As we continue to talk, he demands further connection with me, now insisting that I look into his eyes consistently. I struggle to focus my gaze on him, increasingly aware of my own eyes, drying from lack of blinking. He senses my discomfort as I approach the ultimate topic.

"Joshua . . . dude . . . I have to admit you to the hospital," I say as gently as I can.

"Can't you just be cool?" he begs.

"I can't send a naked growling guy back out onto the streets," I tell him lightly, jokingly. "People would make fun of me. My boss would kill me."

"Let me talk to your boss," he argues. "What's his number? We can call him right now!"

"Joshua, it's two in the morning on a Saturday night. I am not calling my boss at home. Forget my boss. *I* know. You need to be admitted." I have to switch gears. It's lame of me to blame my boss; I have to be the grown-up, be the doctor, and take responsibility for admitting him myself. Being cool cannot be the priority just now.

"You need some help. You need to hang out here and get your head together. It won't be for too long, but you need to check into the hospital for a little break." I point out to him that he is not taking care of himself, and he is endangering himself. His physical health is deteriorating, despite his insistence that he can survive on the streets by eating the free peanuts that the vendors toss him. He is putting himself at risk by arguing with large men on the city streets and parading naked up Broadway. Surely he can see that?

He glares at me, resentful that I have taken this stance. I have crossed back over to the other side, separating and drawing a firm line between us. There is no longer a blurring of boundaries or a flexibility in our roles, and we are no longer confidants. He is the patient, I am the doctor, and I am admitting him involuntarily to the Bellevue psych ward. I am the one with the keys to the unit; he is the one already locked into the detainable area, whether he knows it or not.

"So, you just sit there in judgment of me. You think you can decide who is crazy and who isn't," he says.

I picture myself standing on the corner of Sane and Insane directing traffic. You're in, you're out. Step over the invisible line and see what happens.

"Actually, that is exactly what I do here."

I get up to leave the room. I have more patients to see. I face him and try to smile apologetically as I slowly back out of the door. I assume he won't attack me, but it's always best to err on the side of caution.

Ticket to Ride

When I start my job at Bellevue, in July of 1996, I am a single, thirty-year-old, five-foot-four, pear-shaped gal with long brown hair, freckles, and green eyes. I am smart—more than that, a smart-ass. Growing up in the suburbs of Boston, I got good grades and had plenty of friends. I sported a cool, tough-girl act which served me well over the years. I swore a lot, wore jeans, boots, and a leather vest, and smoked cigarettes. I also played guitar and sang in a rock band.

In high school, I became fascinated by the brain, and by drugs and how they can acutely alter reality, which I discovered via my own travels through the looking glass. I knew I wanted to be a "brain doctor," either a psychiatrist or a neurosurgeon. A premed at Penn, I majored in the Biological Basis of Behavior, devouring coursework in psychology, neurobiology, and psychopharmacology, great training for my eventual career in psychiatry. My cousin was going to Penn Med at the time, and I would run into him around campus. He introduced me to a friend of his who was doing his psychiatry rotation, who was surprised to learn that there was not much emphasis on psychotherapy anymore. "Psychiatry's all pretty much done with medication now," he told me, disheartened, but I was thrilled, looking forward to immersing myself in a prescription-driven field. I was enraptured by the brain and how it could misfire, but it wasn't just the hardware that intrigued me, it was the software with the bugs. And if I was interested in how drugs affected the mind, psychiatry made a lot more sense than neurosurgery.

All through college and medical school, it wasn't enough for me to ace my exams, I had to be the one who turned in the test first, and gave the teacher attitude to boot. Ultracompetitive but trying to look like a slacker, I thought it wouldn't seem cool to try too hard. I studied in the back corner of the library, never letting on that I had to work for my successes.

There was a brief detour in my senior year at Penn, when I decided that I didn't want to become a doctor after all. It was the late 1980s, and I deluded myself into thinking I was the next Madonna, or maybe Chrissie Hynde from the Pretenders. I took a year off after graduation, singing in my band, playing the electric guitar, and riding a motorcycle through the streets of Philadelphia. Even though I had taken my med school exams, filled out all the forms and written the essays, I ended up throwing it all away, literally. I tossed the sealed, addressed envelope containing my application into the garbage the day after my new band formed, sure we were going to make it big, and even more convinced that I had to try. I didn't want to spend the rest of my life wondering about what could have been. My parents were understandably furious.

After a year of playing in the band and working in a Philly hospital doing neurology research, I got bored and decided to get back on track and go to med school, but I didn't quit the band. I spent a good chunk of my first two years at Temple Med going to rehearsals and gigs while studying anatomy and physiology. I crammed for exams in between takes in the recording studio, or sat in my car in the parking lot of a nightclub catching up with my textbooks between the sets of a Saturday night concert.

Eventually I quit the band. Once I started my clinical rotations, there was no time for anything but the hospital and sleep. After graduating from med school, I landed a psychiatric residency at Mount Sinai Hospital in New York City. After that, I ended up at Bellevue. Where all the other crazy people end up.

Psychotic people come to our psych ER from all over the world, as if Bellevue were a beacon, lighting the way. Patients will explain, "I started to hear voices, so I figured I should be at Bellevue." They'll walk from New Jersey, take buses from Missouri, hop flights from Cairo. One woman walked across the George Washington Bridge carrying two large bags full of her own feces, because she somehow knew she needed to be here. (The feces are hard to explain. Some patients, when they become psychotic, collect all sorts of things that take on special meaning for them.)

Bellevue is a full-service hospital in Manhattan, but many assume it is primarily a psychiatric hospital. The police in New York City are guilty of this as well. They will pull people off of the bridges, out of the subway tunnels, or in from the tarmacs of the airports and deliver them straight to us. Even though the public hospitals throughout the city are divided by catchment areas, the cops bring us psychiatric cases from all five boroughs, knowing that we can handle the patients no one else can.

So why am I so attracted to this patient population? I've always been enthralled by insanity. When I was a kid and my parents would take me into Boston, I'd immediately notice the homeless schizophrenics, how they would walk around pelvis-first, talking to themselves. I was fascinated by the idea of hearing voices, of paranoia and disorganized speech. I wanted to understand and help them, but I also think my desire was about wanting to play with fire, to swim in the deep end.

So now I am the doctor in charge of Bellevue's psychiatric emergency room, also known as CPEP (pronounced "See-Pep," the Comprehensive Psychiatric Emergency Program). I run two fifteen-hour overnight shifts on Saturday and Sunday nights. They call me "the weekend attending." It feels just like rock-and-roll psychiatry to me. This is my Saturday night gig.

My work week starts on Saturday evening at six thirty. As I drive south from my apartment near Mount Sinai on the Upper East Side, the East River is on my left, the UN on my right, and I make it to the hospital in about twelve minutes. There is a great view of the Empire State Building as I walk toward the hospital from the back parking lot. I pass the older buildings, the storied repositories for the disenfranchised, which now house the shelters. There are broken statues on the lawn, the grass overgrown behind the wrought iron fences that surround the decrepit buildings. Faded signs point to destinations no longer in existence.

Bellevue is the oldest public hospital in the United States, with a long tradition of "serving the underserved." Its origins date back to a six-bed infirmary which opened in 1736. Bellevue has been an almshouse, a penal institution, and most infamously, an asylum: In 1878, a dedicated pavilion for the insane was christened. The world's first hospital ambulance service, maternity ward, pediatric clinic, and emergency room all got their start right here, but it's the asylum that gets remembered, the ultimate symbol of bedlam that is most strongly yoked to Bellevue's name.

"Take him to Bellevue," is the line I remember best from the old TV cop show *Barney Miller*. It was Hal Linden's answer for any arrestee who was off his rocker. I remember watching that show and wondering, *Where is this magical place?*

I spent my adult life insatiably educating myself on insanity and its treatment, and as soon as I could get a job there, I did.

A Day in the Life

The doors whoosh open automatically as I walk into the ambulance bay by the medical ER, called the AES (for Adult Emergency Services). I say hello to the hospital police officers who are stationed here. Bellevue employs nearly eighty of their own cops, and I get to know all of them over the years as their positions rotate through the various security desks and entrances of the buildings. When there is a ruckus in the psych ER and the staff needs more hands on deck, "HP!" is our SOS. The hospital police hear "HP to CPEP" over their walkie-talkies and come running, stopping briefly to put on a pair of gloves before jumping in to restrain an agitated patient.

The back hallways leading from the AES to the CPEP are interrupted by multiple sets of double doors. Off the hall to the right is the radiology suite, where chest X-rays and CT scans are performed. On the left is "the blue room," the holding area for prisoners who have been treated and released and are waiting for the bus to take them back to Rikers Island. When the prison guards amass a busload on Monday mornings, the prisoners, dressed in orange jumpsuits, their hands and legs shackled, will make their way through these back hallways toward the rear exit, where a bus is idling. It is the most abject, sorrowful group of men you will ever see. They are captive and sick, suffering physically as well as mentally. Many are in withdrawal from whatever was keeping them going on the outside. Others have swallowed taped-up razor blades or lightbulbs in an effort to leave the prison and be admitted to the hospital.

While the procession slowly makes its way toward the back door, two corrections officers at either end hold up the traffic, forcing all the Bellevue staff in the corridor to wait until the prisoners have left. The Rikers inmates march right by the entrance to CPEP. When I first started at Bellevue, I was callous, posturing with bravado while I stood there watching them pass. Sometimes I'd even whistle "I Love a Parade" as they went by. Over the years, my demeanor has softened; now, when the prisoners troop by, I am silent and respectful, offering a sympathetic smile, saying "Hey" if I catch anyone's eye.

Across the hall from the CPEP entrance, there is a suite of offices and call-rooms. Call-rooms are places where doctors can theoretically sleep during the nights they spend "on-call," in the hospital. My first call-room at Bellevue was small and cold, with a rock-hard, narrow bed. When the CPEP moved to its new location, one year after I arrived, I got a larger office. When I got pregnant a few years later, I splurged for a queen-sized bed. It is the largest in the hospital, as far as I know.

As I walk into my call-room, all the way in the back corner of the suite, I throw my things on the bed and check my voice mail before gathering my belongings for the shift. CPEP keys go in the tiny front-right pocket of my jeans; I call this the drug pocket, because it's where patients tend to stash their favorite pills, baggies of dope, or crack vials. My Bellevue ID gets clipped to my scrub top, as does one black pen. My beeper clips to the waistband of my jeans. I grab a water bottle, and my clipboard and folder (stuffed with reference material, like how long cocaine metabolites stay positive in urine samples and how many milligrams of Xanax equal a similar dose of Valium), and head for the door.

My hair is still wet from the shower I took before I left my apartment as I walk through the patient waiting area. On one side of the room, six green leather bucket seats are connected by a metal bar. Above the chairs, pictures of flowers framed in plastic are bolted to the wall.

The hospital police officer assigned to this area sits at a desk with a patient log book. If he's not writing an entry, he may be reading a magazine or watching a portable DVD player, but more likely he is shooting the breeze with a real cop from the NYPD. These guys love to tell war stories, trying to outdo each other with the most outrageous or horrifying narratives.

Once a patient has been logged in by HP and then registered by the clerk, who sits like a bank teller behind Plexiglas, he is sent to see a nurse in the triage room, a windowed cell that separates the patient waiting area from the nurses' station. My own progress through CPEP mirrors the journey the patients take, and I greet the hospital police officer, the clerk, and the triage nurse as I pass each one. I use my key to enter the main area of the psych ER, the locked detainable area, noting the noise, the smell, and the level of activity that will surround me for the next dozen hours or so.

Once I'm in the nurses' station within the locked area, the first thing I need to know to get the ball rolling is the census. How many patients are on hold, admitted, or waiting to be seen? How many of the admissions have been assigned to a bed upstairs and how many will remain in CPEP because the inpatient units have filled up? My biggest concern is back-up on either end. Is the waiting area full of patients yet to be seen, or is the locked detainable area crowded with stalled admissions? Priority one is to keep the census down.

Priority two is to get NYPD out of our waiting area. They have brought their prisoners to be evaluated prior to arraignment, and we need to help make it as brief a detour as possible. Bellevue has a job to do for the city, assisting NYPD in keeping their prisoners safe. Any arrested person who has a psychiatric history or is taking psych meds (this includes the Upper West Side mom on Prozac caught shoplifting) needs to be screened by us. If the police suspect that their prisoner is suicidal, they'll bring him to Bellevue for screening, because it's not safe to leave a potential suicide alone in a cell. Sometimes, a prisoner is so grossly psychotic that it is inappropriate for him to be held in police custody. Ever since one deranged man at central booking—who was never referred for a psych evaluation—stepped on another's neck and killed him, we have been screening more prisoners than ever.

Whenever an arrested person is brought to Bellevue, the job of the psychiatrist is well circumscribed. It is only to ascertain if the patient is calm enough to stand in front of a judge and be arraigned, and whether there is an acute risk of self-harm or danger to others while in police custody. This is called a pre-arraignment evaluation. It is not my responsibility to determine the patient's capacity to stand trial, and it is certainly not my place to judge guilt or innocence.

If a prisoner requires an admission, he is sent to 19 West, the forensic unit. The other inpatient units occupy multiple floors and wings. 20 South is the unlocked detox ward for voluntary patients only. All the other psych wards are locked, even though they house a mixture of voluntary and involuntary patients. 20 East is a dual diagnosis ward for psychiatric patients with alcoholism or drug addiction, the bulk of our clientele. 20 North is the geriatric unit. 18 South has Mandarin- and Cantonese-speaking staff for our Asian immigrant patients. 19 North is the teaching unit for particularly interesting or complicated cases. 12 South is the med/psych unit for those in need of intravenous medication or other intensive medical treatments.

Many of the patients are eligible for more than one unit, but I can only send them up if I know there are empty beds waiting for them. The nurses upstairs don't like new patients coming in over the weekend, so they play games with their own census data, making it seem as though they couldn't possibly take one more patient. Then on Sunday night, sure as the *60 Minutes* clock will tick on CBS, the "mystery beds" miraculously open up, and there is a merciful drainage of our area. The problem is, this relief valve is usually nowhere in sight when I arrive on Saturday night.

But there are other options: I don't have to admit all the patients upstairs. We have our own six-bed ward, the EOU (Extended Observation Unit), where we can place a patient for up to seventy-two hours on a 9.40, an involuntary admission that gives us up to three days to figure out what's going on with the patient, which ideally involves speaking to family members, employers, and therapists. During their stay, we can see if there's any change in presenting symptoms. Once the time is up, we need to either discharge or admit. We can admit by using either a 9.39, an involuntary admission, or if the patient is willing to sign in voluntarily, a 9.13. All the "9 point something"s require a set of New York State legal papers to be placed in the chart.

If I'm not sure where to place a patient, I have an easy out—a twenty-four-hour Hold requires no legal status, no justification for detainment. Patients spend the night and are reinterviewed in the morning when they're less drunk, high, or sedated. The Hold is the disposition of last resort. It is better for patients to have a definitive status, but sometimes, when they can't give any coherent information, that's impossible. The patients who are safe to be discharged from the CPEP are the T & R's: They are treated and released. They're not sick or dangerous enough to keep hospitalized, so we patch them up and send them back to the front, just like they did on *M*A*S*H,* only our war zone is the mean streets of New York.

Sometimes patients are eager to leave, but other times they mostly want a place to sleep. Occasionally they'll ask earnestly if they can please just spend the night; other times they'll manufacture symptoms in order to dupe me. Either way, I utter my well-rehearsed line, "This isn't a shelter, it's a hospital; you need to be genuinely sick to stay here." The Bellevue men's shelter is just one block north, and many of our discharged patients are referred there, though they are loath to go.

There's an oddball category of patients with no official status that I call "Waiting for Laces." This is a T & R whose discharge paperwork is still pending, sitting in the nondetainable area waiting to speak with a social worker about what we call the "dispo plan"—where to go next and how to follow up with outpatient services. It's a tense, vulnerable position to be in, having been judged sane enough to leave the hospital, but still in limbo while you wait for your walking papers and your belt, shoelaces, and wallet, knowing you need to stay calm and polite in order to be released. Some of these patients are furious at being discharged. They would rather be admitted to Bellevue than sleep on the steaming sidewalk grates or in the subways or shelters. Sometimes they'll make a scene, threatening the staff and requiring hospital police to escort them off the grounds, perhaps without all of their belongings. (When I see the laceless walking the streets of the city, I wonder if they are people who got tired of waiting for the social worker and just left without picking up their belongings, or if they were never actually deemed safe to be discharged but have somehow managed to escape.)

After I have figured out how many patients are in the CPEP and where they're likely to end up, I see how the staffing looks. Do I have any medical students rotating through here tonight? How many residents are here, and are they first-years or second-, slackers or stars? Most important is which attending—which doctor in charge—has been working the shift that immediately precedes mine. This will establish whether I have a mess to clean up or whether things have been left in pretty good shape. Sign-out is the changing of the guard between the attendings. It will occur whenever the departing doctor has the time to sit down and run the list, discussing every patient in the area. Often, there are many loose ends to tie up before that can happen.

A busy Saturday night for me is twenty-five or more patients in the CPEP, or more than five on triage. If there are a lot of triages, I won't wait for sign-out. I will just "glove up and dig in," as they say in medicine. (This saying is medical jargon for manually dis-impacting a constipated patient, but it has morphed into meaning "suck it up and get to work.") I will grab a chart and see any patient who has already been triaged by a nurse and looks like he could be a quick T & R, which only involves writing up the interview and a discharge order, considerably less paperwork than the other dispo plans, since there are no legal forms or admission orders to fill out.

When it is less busy, the first order of business is, "When's dinner and where are we ordering from?" This was especially true during the months at Bellevue when I happened to be pregnant and took "eating for two" very seriously.

The nights tend to progress smoothly. The on-call resident and medical students see the triages, and then present the cases to me. I help them decide who stays and who goes, and I check over all the paperwork to make sure the admissions get packaged for transfer to the upstairs wards. By one a.m., I usually turn in, letting the resident run the show in my absence. I am available for phone calls and consultations, both by the second-year resident in the CPEP and the third-year who is doing consultations upstairs in the rest of the hospital. The attendings in the medical ER often call me as well, to let me know they're sending someone over to CPEP. I usually sleep about five hours or so, though it is interrupted by multiple phone calls, and occasionally I need to go across the hall to deal with some problem or fill out restraint orders that require an attending's signature.

I don't usually eat like a lumberjack, but on Sunday mornings I make an exception. It's the middle of my Bellevue weekend, and I like to treat myself. Short stack, two eggs over easy on the side, sausage split. I've developed little traditions as the years have gone by, and the men behind the counter at the Bellevue coffee shop, with their easy grins and mischievous eyes, have kept up with my preferences. Their pancakes are legendary among the ambulance drivers and police officers, and their prices are so low even the panhandlers can sit down to a good meal.

I bring my breakfast back to the CPEP and give sign-out to the Sunday morning attending and the moonlighting residents hired to work the weekend day shift. By ten, I am out the door for my eight hours off before I drive back into work Sunday night and do it all over again.

Hello Goodbye

M y oatmeal with sliced banana and my lousy Bellevue coffee are lined up in front of me on the counter of the nurses' station. I spend a few minutes opening and sprinkling the sugar packets into the two matching paper cups, one filled with brown liquid, the other with brown solid, waiting for the other doctors, psychology interns, and social workers to arrive. The crowd assembles, the nurses are called over to join us, and it's a little after 8:30 when the CPEP director instructs me to begin the Monday morning sign-out. It's time for me to download what I've been doing all weekend and who's still left in the area.

Mostly what I've been doing is trying to stem the tide of patients flowing into CPEP. When there's a slew of patients on triage and no empty beds upstairs, I can call my own 911, the EMS diversion desk, and beg them to take us out of the loop. It's a number I know by heart already. An EMS is quick to remind me, diversion is a courtesy. They can make an announcement to all the ambulances, telling them we're full to the brim, but they can't guarantee compliance. And once an ambulance shows up, I can't turn them away. And the walk-ins are still going to come regardless of our diversion status, so there's only so much I can do to relieve the pressure of the incoming patients on the area.

I begin morning report with an announcement. "Listen up. We're on diversion, confirmed by EMS operator 8758. It's good till noon, for what it's worth. Okay, here we go. Starting with the voluntary admissions, on a 9.13 is Mr. R. He's a fifty-two-year-old African-American male with a history of schizophrenia and alcohol abuse, and he's hep C positive. He walked in Saturday night saying he'll kill the person at the shelter who stole his meds and wallet. He's got a history of aggressive behavior, though nothing recent. Also, he did a stint at the Greenhouse drug rehab program not too long ago. He's on Zyprexa for his psychotic symptoms and behavioral control, and a Librium taper for the alcohol withdrawal. Keep an eye on his vital signs. Also, rule out malingering. He could be faking it, just looking for a better place to crash, and the homicidal threats are bogus.

"Then there's Mr. J, thirty-five-year-old Hispanic guy, also with schizophrenia, who was referred from the walk-in clinic on Friday. He's been noncompliant with his outpatient treatment, showing up sporadically, going on and off his meds. He's getting delusional, says he's going to confront people with tattoos and piercings because they are in league with Satan. That should keep him busy for a while. He's on Risperdal one milligram twice a day.

"Moving on to the involuntaries, Ms. D is a fifty-three-year-old black female brought in by EMS from the Port of Atrocities Bus Terminal on Saturday morning, where she threw a fit because she felt that someone had touched her. She was almost arrested, but once the cops got a sense of her, they decided to make her an EDP so they could just drop her off here instead of taking her downtown and booking her. They made the right choice, actually. She's pretty intense, irritable, paranoid, disorganized. She came with a notebook full of stuff about the Devil and God doing battle inside her, that sort of thing. She denies a psych history, but she looks like a street schiz. Also, she's got a history of cardiac issues, hypertension, chest pain. She needs blood pressure meds written before she goes upstairs.

"Mr. S is a thirty-six-year-old Hispanic man with a history of depression who currently lives with his sister and is unemployed. He recently returned from Puerto Rico with worsening depression. He banged his head repeatedly against a wall in a suicide attempt on Saturday, got bandaged up in the AES Saturday night, and then started head-banging here, too. Head CT is clear; he's neurologically intact. His utox is positive for cocaine. His ex-wife says he's been depressed for years and he acts out whenever they have a fight, which they did recently in PR. He seemed calmer on Sunday, but he was pretty agitated on Saturday. He's on Lexapro for the depression, and prn Librium as needed. He's a drinker. No signs of withdrawal so far, so we haven't given him any, but keep an eye on his vitals.

"Mr. A is a twenty-four-year-old black male brought in by EMS on Sunday afternoon. He approached the MTA police asking to be placed in a witness protection program. He's got elaborate paranoid delusions involving kidnapping, murder, being followed. . . . He's denying all psych history and all psych symptoms; the only thing he'll cop to is that he hasn't slept in three nights. He's been pretty wired in here. He thinks the TV is sending him messages and that the news has to do with him. We have him on Risperdal one milligram twice a day."

I detail the arrival, diagnosis, and management of another dozen involuntary admissions, before adding, "One more admission: Mr. H is a twenty-three-year-old Hispanic male with a history of bipolar disorder. His mom is too, by the way, so easy when you talk to her on the phone—she sounds pretty manic herself; she's talking a mile a minute and it's pretty hard to follow. The patient was brought in by EMS on Sunday afternoon after he approached NYPD on the street, asking to go to the hospital. He was complaining of anxiety, suicidal thoughts, and paranoia to the cops, but here he's denying everything. He looks intense, guarded, and he may be responding to internal stimuli. He denies alcohol and drugs. Anyway, last week he took a handful of his mood stabilizer Depakote in a suicide attempt, but he never sought any medical attention. His friend says he was talking about throwing himself in front of a bus for the past couple of days. We're waiting on Tylenol and aspirin levels just to make sure, but he looks okay medically. He should be on Risperdal and Depakote once the labs come back. Can somebody check those and write the orders?

"Okay, in the EOU we have three admissions. I left some room in there for you guys. Bachelor number one is a thirty-eight-year-old black male . . . well, she's a transsexual actually. Okay, bachelorette number one walked in claiming she was raped but was really disorganized and out of it, and at one point she told AES she lied about the rape to get a place to sleep. She was grossly psychotic and definitely high on cocaine. That was Saturday night. On Sunday, she was irritable, still pretty disorganized, and insisting we give her housing. The plan is to discharge today if she's cleared. If she's not, give her a bed upstairs. A single if possible.

"EOU bed two is a forty-two-year-old black male with schizophrenia and AIDS. He was brought in by EMS from his adult home, saying the voices were telling him to hurt someone and he didn't want to. He's compliant with Zyprexa, and a second antipsychotic, Geodon, and his HIV meds. We're hoping a short stay in the bed and breakfast suite will take the voices down a notch. He just came in last night so give him some time to pull it together. He's a nice guy, actually—genuinely ill and pretty mild-mannered. Wouldn't hurt a flea, I bet.

"EOU bed three is Mr. G. He's a twenty-year-old Hispanic man brought in by EMS Saturday morning. He came here by bus from Massachusetts to meet Wu Tang Clan. He says he's a famous rapper himself and he has four jobs. Totally grandiose, bizarre, tangential, poor boundaries. He'll need a bed upstairs for sure, but we're keeping him in the EOU because he's all over the place and needs his own room. Also, we're pretty backed up; the admissions aren't going anywhere soon, so he'll need to have his status changed to 9.39 sometime today or tomorrow, when his EOU time runs out. Spoke to mom who says he was doing okay on Risperdal and Depakote, but he's probably gone off his meds, so we restarted them.

"On Hold is Mr. W, a seventeen-year-old white male with a history of bipolar. He was brought in by EMS Sunday night from home after throwing some furniture around and getting pretty violent. He's got a solid history given his age, multiple med trials, multiple psych hospitalizations. He just got out of Saint Vinnie's a couple of weeks ago. He was pretty combative when he first got here, tore up the peds ER pretty good last night, but once we got some prn's in him, he calmed down. He's been pacing up a storm, can't really sit still. He may have akathisia from recent med switches so we're holding the antipsychotics for right now. Child psych is supposed to see him this morning.

"But wait! There's more!" I say like I'm selling something on TV. "There's a few on triage. I'm sorry. They just rolled in this morning. One guy, a prisoner, Mr. K, forty-eight-year-old guy arrested for robbery, just got out of Rikers a week ago. He says he takes Risperdal and Sinequan for sleep. He's asking for a few sandwiches and then he says he can go to arraignment. He's an easy T & R.

"Also on triage is Mr. U, a thirty-eight-year-old Indian man who walked in this morning. Looks very well groomed and also very tense. Complains of feeling electric shocks in his head. Somebody make sure he's not going through Effexor withdrawal. He's preoccupied with religion, changing from Jewish to Muslim to Christian in the course of a quick conversation with the clerk during registration.

"And, last but not least, Unknown Black Male, looks to be in his thirties, sent from Coney Island Hospital, arrested for assaulting an MTA worker with a cane. Whose cane I do not know. Not his. He got IM'd with all kinds of sedation at Coney and is totally shlogged. Apparently he was very combative there, and was also spitting at the staff. They called me about the transfer last night but he hadn't been medically cleared yet. They have very little info on him and NYPD is going to run a missing persons. He was pretty violent at Coney; he needed four cops to escort him here, so be careful when he wakes up.

"Okay, that's all I got. I'm outta here. Have a good week, you guys." I gather my folder and water bottle and leave the nurses' station. "Enjoy!"

In the nondetainable area, EMS is bringing in another case as I walk out.

"We're on diversion," I say as I head for the exit.

"Oh, really? No one told us that," answers the driver.

But I keep right on walking, because my shift is done. It's someone else's problem now.

My life at Bellevue happens in spurts, in weekly installments like episodes of a dramatic series. I have all week off to recover and to process whatever's gone down. Like a woman after childbirth, I forget the pain. I come home Monday morning wired and fried, but by Saturday evening, I'm showered in a freshly laundered scrub top, ready to take sign-out.

Girl

(Temple Medical School, Philadelphia, 1988)

Looking back on it, I remember the first year of medical school as cycles of filling and then emptying my head: reading, memorizing, cramming for tests, regurgitating all I had learned, and then, in most cases, immediately forgetting it. It was, in many ways, like being brainwashed. I learned a completely new language, and it insidiously changed my perception. One day I was in the library studying, gazing at the signs on the shelves, and I was so immersed in that new language that I misread the sign that said "periodicals" as "pericardial"—that being the word for the sac that surrounds the heart. I walked around Philadelphia looking at its inhabitants not as citizens, but as patients. That guy with the limp and the drooping face must've had a stroke. This one with the tremor and the stooped posture's got Parkinson's disease. Everywhere, instead of people, I saw pathology. I was learning to think like a doctor.

I would study so much, I'd feel like the information was going to leak out of my ears. By the summer between my first and second years, I felt I needed a break from studying. I wanted to be around patients, preferably crazy ones. My search for a job brought me to a hallway outside the locked psych ward of Temple Hospital, where I sat waiting to meet with a psychologist who was doing research on auditory hallucinations. I had my motorcycle helmet with me, and my backpack. A slave to eighties fashion, I wore a green-flowered jumper with black leggings and black wrestling boots. My hair was styled in a spiky crew cut with a foot-long braided tail, tied at the end with a white bow. I must've looked like a freak to the psychologist, but after a short chat, he hired me to help him interview one hundred hallucinating patients— a dream job for me, though it paid nothing.

I wandered the psych wards for the next several months, making friends with the psychotic patients so we could get our data. It was great fun, a true pleasure to be learning more about my chosen field well ahead of schedule, and a welcome respite from reading. I hung out in the patient's lounge, smoking cigarettes with the patients in an effort to ingratiate myself into their cliques. There was one tall, thin man who stayed for months, waiting for a state hospital bed. He had tried to cut off his penis, explaining to me that he felt it was the root of all evil; he joked with me that he would call his memoir *Woody*. There were many afternoons when he'd wander the hallways singing the lyrics to "Right Here Waiting": "Oceans apart, day after day, and I slowly go insane." I'd join him on the chorus, adding harmony to his plaintive voice. "Wherever you go, whatever you do, I will be right here waiting for you," as if assuring him he'd always be able to come back to me on the inpatient ward if he couldn't make it on the outside.

The research project inched forward as I recruited new hallucinating patients into our study, running the interviews in a small room down the hall from the locked unit. In between, I attended the weekly staff meetings to discuss the patients. We gathered around a huge conference table: the doctors and nurses in charge of the two units, the chief resident, and me. I was the youngest in the room. The head of the acute ward was a short, playful doctor who moved the meetings along, peppering his descriptions of patients with words like "bonkers" and "bananas." He obviously loved the patients and his job, but he called it like it was. He taught me that it was okay to marvel at the madness, to be titillated by the sheer lunacy that waited to envelop me on the wards. Also, he was clearly enamored with the chief resident, Lucy, a gal from Georgia with a strident Southern accent. She had light brown hair that wildly pointed this way and that, and she always seemed to be wearing a Hawaiian shirt, or something so bright and flowery that it should only be worn on an island. She was the most charismatic doctor I had come across in my training, and I wanted to be just like her when I grew up. In the staff meetings she was irreverent, flippant, and hilarious. The older doctors treated her as a prodigal genius-rebel. They put up with her sass, laughing in spite of themselves. In the hallways with her peers, or on the wards among the patients, she strutted with a swagger in her walk, captivating all in her path with her broad, knowing grin, her bravado, and her down-home charm.

After several months on the wards, I asked my boss if I could hang out in the psych ER one night, knowing it was a night that Lucy was on-call. I spent the hours before the shift making homemade wontons in my cramped kitchen, mincing the garlic and water chestnuts, grating the carrots and ginger.

It was cold and rainy as I drove my beat-up Honda Civic to Temple's psych ER. When I finally tracked down the good doctor, she was in an office with her feet up, wearing her usual button-down Hawaiian shirt over her scrubs, her hair all akimbo. "Slow night tonight," she apologized. "You may not get to see much."

"I brought you some wontons. Actually, they're Korean. They're called *mondu*," I told her, fishing them out of my bag. "I thought you might be hungry."

"You're kidding me. You *made* these?"

I felt foolish, like a kindergartner who'd brought an apple for the teacher, except that this apple took two and a half hours to create.

The ER was dead as promised. We saw no patients together, but we chatted about my plans for a future in psychiatry, and I gushed over how much it excited me—the patients, their symptoms and stories, the pharmacology. We bonded over our love of psychosis, how easily we found ourselves mesmerized by the potency of insanity. She told me war stories about her training, the kinds of patients who impressed her, and what she did to make an equal impression on them. Her boasting was engaging and endearing, and I was treated to an outpouring of tales about her rebellious adolescence and college years: how she worked construction and drove a backhoe one summer, how she called her father's bosses "assholes" when unknowingly on speakerphone in his office, the time she got drunk in medical school and "beat up a car." I noticed her boundaries were very loose, like mine, and she didn't censor herself when regaling me with her greatest hits. Our styles were similar, and I had a feeling that she learned to act macho as a young girl to win the approval of her father, just as I had done.

Although I was only a medical student, she treated me as an equal,

taking me into her confidence, telling me about things I didn't necessarily have a right to hear, like the leather fetish of one of the Temple
psychiatrists. With this segue, she mentioned that she was a lesbian.

I was speechless.

For some reason, this had not occurred to me. I thought we were
alike. I identified with her so strongly, wanting to be just like her. And
she was gay? What did that say about me, with some sort of schoolgirl crush on her? I had to say something quickly, or there would be an
uncomfortable silence and I would look like an idiot.

"Do your parents know?" I stammered, transforming myself into a
twelve-year-old girl from Kansas.

"Of course!" she answered, irritated, dismissive, confirming my fears.
Our conversation died. She clearly thought I was a boob. I left shortly
afterwards, mortified at fumbling the most basic of exchanges. I wanted
her to befriend me, to take me under her wing, but I was sure I'd ruined
any chance of that.

Another Girl

The initial two years of med school are known as the "preclinical" years. We learned anatomy from dead bodies, and we pored over thick, heavy books filled with disgusting pictures. The tail end of the second year was spent getting the medical students more comfortable with the idea of patient contact. The faculty cautiously introduced us onto the wards to take histories from inpatients.

When I finally got to practice interviewing a real live human, the woman I'd been assigned to had the chills and was coughing. It was unsettling to sit so close to her. All my life I'd been told to keep my distance from anyone who was ill and possibly contagious. "What the hell am I doing near this sick person?" the medical students joked with each other when we met up at the bar later.

The first time I ever performed a gynecological exam, it was with a paid model. I was in a room with two other medical students, both men—big, hulking jocks actually—shaking with fear, stinking up the small exam room with their acrid sweat. (There are two types of sweat: the more watery kind, eccrine, that results from overheating, and the hormone-laden kind, apocrine, that comes from terror. Fear sweat smells a whole lot worse than exercise sweat.) When the teaching attending came in and asked who would go first, the two men looked at me wide-eyed, silently pleading. I volunteered to go first, and the model could not have been any nicer.

"If you are commenting on appearances during the exam, use words like 'normal' and 'healthy,' " advised the professor.

"I guess 'Nice rack' doesn't go over so well, huh?" I joked nervously. No one else thought this was funny, including me. My mouth was dry, my insides trembling, and I felt utterly alone. I performed the breast exam, feeling for lumps, and the vaginal exam, feeling for ovaries, as best I could, and then it was time to insert the speculum. I was supposed to slide it in closed, then open it up once it was inside the vagina. My big gaffe, which I'm sure was profoundly uncomfortable for the model, was that I removed the speculum without closing it first. I realized that I'd hurt her, and felt like a buffoon. As I apologized profusely, she was kind and sincere, understanding my mortification. (I still remember her to this day, and would again like to apologize and thank her for not yelling at me. I would've yelled.)

Every July first is New Year's Day for medical students—the first day of the new academic year. Recently graduated medical students become "doctors," and second-year medical students become the much anticipated "third-years," when the clinical rotations begin. No more lecture halls; it's finally time to learn on patients.

And so, in the summer of 1990, things finally got interesting. I left the classrooms, the endless labs, and the solitary studying. It was time for me to enter the hospital, and it was baptism by fire: I was assigned to surgery. I knew nothing—nothing practical, that is, nothing of any use to a surgeon. I didn't know how to draw blood. I didn't know how to order medications or labs, or how to check the lab results, or even where the lab was. I was worse than useless: I was a burden, plagued by the constant anxiety of "I've never done this before."

But the surgery residents had been where we were, and they knew the deal. They were used to teaching clueless kids in July. They knew the best patients for teaching were those who could not complain. At Albert Einstein hospital in the heart of Northern Philadelphia, that meant either a patient who was unconscious or was simply unaware that they could've asked for someone other than a medical student to provide their care.

A tremendously obese woman was brought into the emergency

room by her family because of some sort of a boil on her belly. The cyst was enormous and angry red, with striations of scarlet spidering off its center. The patient was feverish and somnolent from the infection, which we would later diagnose as necrotizing fasciitis, requiring multiple surgeries to "debride" or remove the infected tissue. She was put on oxygen and given something for the pain, and then we swarmed in like ants on a melon rind. Her blood needed to be drawn, her cyst fluid to be cultured. She also required an arterial blood gas, an exquisitely painful procedure where a needle is inserted into an artery, as opposed to the standard venous draw adequate for most blood work. The surgery resident showed a group of us how to locate the artery by feeling the pulse prior to inserting the needle. Since this woman was nearly comatose, she wouldn't mind if I didn't get it on my first try. I was surprised to see that my hands had a fine tremor as I fished around for the artery. (When I attempted this on a conscious patient the next day, he winced stoically at first, then eventually tore his arm away, screaming and swearing at me, and I had to enter into complex negotiations with him for cooperation.)

Taking a history to establish what was wrong with a patient was much trickier than cramming for exams. They didn't know the names or dosages of their medications. They pronounced their diagnoses in a way that confounded me as to what they actually had. A patient told me she was just getting over her "flea bites" which, after some detective work, turned out to be phlebitis. Another man reported he was taking "peanut butter balls" for his seizures. The ER docs had a good laugh over this, translating "phenobarbital" for me. When I asked a patient, "Where were you shot?" I got aggravated when he answered, "Right down on Broad Street," which is the information his friends might've appreciated. I, on the other hand, needed to know where on his body. Misunderstandings like these abounded. (The classic medical school joke is to ask a patient if she's sexually active, to which she will reply, "No, I usually just lie there.")

My surgery rotation was part ER, part surgical wards, and part operating room. I developed a love-hate relationship with the adrenaline and the hours. I would repeatedly envision Hawkeye Pierce (this was before *Grey's Anatomy*) each time I scrubbed-in at the sink with the other surgeons and then pushed my back through the OR door, my arms at ninety-degree angles. I spent most of my time feeling like I was in either a gory movie or a well-written medical drama. *I am playing the part of a doctor,* I told myself, *and hopefully, eventually, I will feel like one.*

Philadelphia in July was a festival of mortality: car accidents, gunshot wounds, stabbings, muggings. A man with his initials in gold on his top two teeth stumbled into the ER literally holding his guts. He had been shot in the belly and his intestines had "avulsed" outside of his skin. I was invited to join in his surgery. Instead of using a scalpel to open his abdomen, they used the bovie, the device typically used to cauterize bleeders, something like a hot poker. As the surgery commenced, there was a small explosion as the escaped intestinal gas ignited the bovie. "Okay, that means he's perfed his intestines somewhere," the resident explained to me calmly, in contrast to my jumpiness. We examined what seemed like miles of his intestines, passing them through our hands trying to find the perforation. He had been shot with a shotgun, and the chief resident made the same joke repeatedly as he dropped endless pieces of buckshot into a silver bowl held by the nurse. "Send this to ballistics," he quipped as one clinked. "This one too." "Ballistics." He thought it would never get old, and for some reason, he was right. It's all in the delivery.

It was during these first few months of my third year that I learned something crucial about myself: I couldn't stand to see people writhing in pain. I felt horrible that they were suffering and I wasn't yet in any position to stop it. Broken bones sticking out of skin or fractures grinding against themselves when the limb was moved (a sound called crepitus) creeped me out more than anything. But give me someone in psychic pain, whose soul was aching, and I felt fully equipped to involve myself.

The surgical residents sensed this in me, and I was frequently pulled along when one of them had to deliver bad news to a patient or family member.

On the Fourth of July weekend I was helping to cover the ER. I was very excited, and a bit nervous, because a trauma call had come in. EMS was five minutes out, bringing us someone from a car accident. The members of the trauma team converged on the ER from various parts of the hospital—the surgeon's lounge, the wards, the call-room. We "gowned up" in yellow plastic robes, gloves, and goggles. We were gathered around a gurney waiting for the ambulance when I heard the chief surgeon of the trauma team say, "Remember, it's not a trauma call, it's a trauma code." I had no idea what the difference was but I stayed mum as she explained to the third-year resident, "She's already coded. All we can do is try to revive her."

I realized then that we were all dressed up and waiting for a dead girl.

When EMS wheeled the patient in, they gave their report. "Sixteen-year-old girl, unknown medical history, unrestrained, driving a Suzuki Samurai which flipped multiple times. She was thrown from the car. CPR started in the field." As she was transferred from the ambulance stretcher to our gurney, I noticed her small, light-blue running shoes, the razor stubble on her legs, her turquoise terry-cloth shorts, and her chipped fingernail polish.

We began our efforts at resuscitation. Her eyes were open and staring at the ceiling as her clothes were cut from her body. A male nurse noticed she was wearing contact lenses and removed them, telling me how her eyes would dry out if we left them in. The girl did not blink.

"You see that? Not good," the nurse explained to me. "She's got no corneal reflexes." I stood by the gurney, trying to make myself small and not get in anyone's way as the doctors and nurses buzzed around the young girl. They put intravenous lines in her arms, a catheter into her bladder, and they checked her for internal bleeding. This is done by peritoneal lavage, which is basically a way to rinse out the inside of the torso. It's not exactly rocket science: If the liquid comes back red, there is internal bleeding. The liquid came back clear. Her heart started beating somehow, but she did not breathe on her own, and so she was intubated and connected to a respirator.

I had been working with a second-year surgical resident up on the wards, and he startled me out of my glassy stare, which mirrored the young girl's.

"Julie. We gotta go talk to the family." As we walked out of the trauma room, I glanced at the small blue sneaker lying on its side in the corner.

These past couple of days, the second-year had seemed like such a softie, apologizing to patients if he needed to draw a blood gas, feeling sorry for a little boy who needed his IV site "cut down," but he hardened up when confronted with this girl's family. As he explained her current condition, I saw him become emotionally removed and overly technical with them—the mother, father, and older sister of a girl who was celebrating her new license to drive. He hid behind the medical jargon, stiffening visibly as he explained our attempts at resuscitation, the condition of the heart, the lungs, the brain, which ones were working now and which weren't. The sister looked at me with such hate in her eyes. Why was she blaming me? I wasn't the doctor delivering the horrible news. But I knew why she was angry. There was something callous and hurtful about his attitude—and therefore mine, by association, although I remained silent, careful not to show any expression—as he catalogued the damage and explained the unlikelihood of her awakening from this coma.

The family insisted that she remain on life support. They had heard of people waking up from comas, they'd seen it on television, and so we were unable to convince them of its improbability. She was admitted to the surgical ICU, a girl with a beating heart and nothing more, taking up an intensive-care bed in the hospital for thousands of dollars a day, so the family could have some time to say good-bye. They were angry and confused, and they wouldn't be rushed into accepting what even I could clearly see: She was gone already.

For reasons I did not yet understand, I ended up displaying the same condescending, remote attitude as my surgical resident when I was asked to go explain her condition again, this time to her high school friends who had gathered in the waiting room: "Right now, your friend is on a machine to keep her alive, and we're not sure she's going to pull through." Short and sweet, and the young girls shrieked and sobbed. They barely stayed to hear my explanation of the shutdown of her various organ systems, turning away to hug each other and cry instead. It was my first time telling anyone their friend was dead, or as good as dead, and my delivery needed work, but doing a surgery rotation in an inner-city hospital would give me plenty of opportunities.

Back at the hospital a few days later, a patient I'd been working with that holiday weekend had tested negative for the AIDS virus. Since I had stuck myself with a needle filled with her blood, I had been anxious, waiting for the results. Unfortunately for the patient, however, the good news about her test results meant very little in the scheme of things. Before the long weekend, she had been hit by a car and had broken her leg. When she left the hospital, with a cast from toes to thigh, she went home to hang out with friends, who, like herself, smoked crack. She must have gone on some sort of a binge; when she eventually started paying attention to her surroundings and her body, she realized that her leg was bothering her. She felt a tingling, an aching, and returned to the ER to have it examined, where she was told she had gangrene in her toes and foot. The cast was too tight and had cut off her circulation.

I was with her, avoiding her eyes and instead staring at her swollen, black toes, when the surgeons gave her the devastating news: She needed an amputation. I spent time with her, helping her to adjust, and was present in the operating room when the lower part of her leg was removed, the electric saw sparing her knee. (For years after this surgery rotation, it was hard for me to eat chicken, turkey, and especially leg of lamb without thinking about amputations.)

On the day when I got the HIV test results back, I rushed to her room to share with her the good news, but I knew the only news she really wanted to hear was that this had all been a bad dream, and things could go back to the way they were when she had two legs. I left her room and walked down the long, windowed hallway that connected the surgery wards to the ICU. I was thrilled she was HIV negative and I didn't have to take AZT, getting tested every few months to see if I "sero-converted," the medical terminology for testing positive. But I couldn't shake the guilt of being the healthy one.

On my way to the elevator, I heard a sound I couldn't immediately identify coming from the ICU. It was a screeching, squealing sound, which stopped to take a breath and returned as a wailing, then a moaning.

The dead girl.

She was scheduled to be taken off her life support that day, after three EEGs had confirmed brain death. It was her mother or her grandmother or her sister who was mourning in a way that I could feel in my gut.

I stood in the hallway by the elevators, unable to press the button that would take me home.

Think for Yourself
(Residency, Mount Sinai Hospital, NYC, 1992)

Fresh out of medical school, I was finally able to call myself doctor. I left Philly and moved to New York to begin my residency in psychiatry. On my first day on the inpatient wards at Mount Sinai Hospital, I walked into my patient's room to introduce myself. He was sitting on his bed, cross-legged, his eyes shining.

"Uh, hello, I'm Doctor Holland," I said awkwardly, not knowing where else to begin.

"Hello, Doctor Holland," he boomed, smiling beatifically. "I . . . am . . . God." He was perched on his bed like a guru on a mountaintop, in the midst of a manic episode, flying high on his own neurochemicals. He felt so good, he squirmed with pleasure, yet his manner was composed, a king on a throne. I called my mother that evening as soon as I walked into my new apartment. My white coat—stuffed with reflex hammer, penlight, and pocket guides—clunked to the floor. "You're not going to believe this. It's the best-case scenario. I am starting my medical career at the very top." I paused for dramatic effect. "I am God's doctor!"

"There's nowhere to go but down," my mother deadpanned.

I hadn't thought of it that way.

I spent my first two years at Mount Sinai treating all kinds of psychiatric patients. I went to weekly lectures and read journal articles to learn more about schizophrenia, Alzheimer's disease, delirium, and Huntington's chorea (a tormenting neurological illness that causes wildly flaying limbs, except in sleep when they mysteriously become still). My patients listened to their voices, talked to themselves, smoked incessantly, urinated on the floors, twitched, shuffled, threatened suicide, and shouted their demands. I conjured up combinations of pharmaceuticals, prepped them for electroshock therapy, performed lumbar punctures, drew blood, and documented everything that happened in their charts. I made multiple diagnoses, managed a slew of medications, explained symptoms to families, and set up clinic appointments prior to discharge.

Some nights I was on call overnight at Mount Sinai Hospital, a few blocks from my Upper East Side apartment; other nights I was at Sinai's other training site, the Veteran's Hospital in the Bronx. There, in the middle of nowhere, I had complete autonomy. I was the only psychiatrist in the house. Frequently, a vet who called himself Morris would call the hospital to speak with the shrink on duty. His calls were legendary—the other residents throughout the city knew about him—and they were a rite of passage for us all. He kept us on the phone as long as he could, asking questions that could not be answered to his satisfaction. "Doc, why do people bless me when I sneeze? What does it mean to fall for someone?" Meanwhile, my pager would go off because someone on the wards had just fallen and cut his head. When I went to examine the patient and order a head CT, there would be a powerful minty-freshness coming from his pores. Mouthwash drunk. Another one. The VA had a store in the lobby that sold toiletries including mouthwash with alcohol, about fifty proof. Vets getting mouthwash-drunk was a rite of passage as inexorable as Morris's calls.

On the wards at Mount Sinai, there was one demented woman in her seventies with long, curly hair dyed Hollywood-blond. She thought I was her daughter and I let her. It was easier for both of us that way. Most days, she was in a lounge chair in front of the nurse's station, secured with something like an apron, so she couldn't slide onto the floor. Her frontal lobes, the parts of the brain that inhibit proscribed behaviors, were shot. She said what was on her mind, which nearly every day, all day, sounded like this: "You look good to me! You look good to me! I want to sex you up, and you, and you!" The more primitive parts of her brain were in charge of her behavior now. Her most elemental desires were gratified with no compunction, no superego to get in the way. On a regular basis, she could be seen masturbating with her free hand, then moaning as she climaxed, and then peeing, her urine pooling on the floor beneath her chair, after which she fell asleep, sated, with a Mona Lisa smile.

"When I go, I wanna go like that," I said to the other doctors.

One of the psych residents I got to know was a guy named Daniel. He was a year ahead of me, and charmingly, dashingly handsome. When he flashed his perfectly straight teeth in a sparkling smile, his cheeks practically eclipsed his eyes. We hung out with the same crowd and saw each other socially a bit, but there was one day on the wards that tried our early friendship. I noticed that his patient—slumped over in a chair, drooling and sleeping deeply—seemed excessively sedated. This is a common situation on the wards. I reviewed her medication list and discussed with the nurses which ones to stop, but she wasn't my patient, she was Daniel's. I was a first-year and he was a second. I had broken the chain of command, disrupting the hierarchy that is the backbone of a teaching hospital. I just thought, *There's a patient who's been overmedicated, what can I do to help?* But it turned out that I stepped on his toes and he did not take it well. As he rebuked me, I saw a side of him I didn't ever want to see again, and what I had seen informed the rest of my interactions with him as my residency progressed. I had to remember to defer to him, which wasn't easy for me. I also had to remember that even though I felt like a pro, I was new at this and had to act accordingly.

All the residents were assigned to a supervisor to help us make sense of all we were going through. Mine was an older gentleman with hearing aids and a perpetually benevolent mien. My toughest case was a gal who kept slapping herself and swearing loudly. She had obsessive-compulsive disorder and Tourette's. She playfully called me Dr. Hollandaise, which my supervisor, an analyst, interpreted for me in a Freudian framework.

"She wants to eat you up. You're saucy and delectable."

Okay, then.

Sarah stayed in her bed most days. She'd wet the bed and not bother to leave it, something that disturbed me inordinately since we were nearly the same age. She was tall, with a humongous head, her face covered in acne. Her big, fleshy lips opened to allow a gruff, insistent voice to escape. She'd bark out swears and racial slurs, then quickly offer her sincere apologies.

I played backgammon with her in the patient lounge when I'd stay late to take call overnight; she had to tap the board and the wall a certain number of times prior to rolling the dice. As the game progressed, her rituals got more complicated until they included her tapping me. She had to touch my arm before she could take her turn. "It's my OCD," she explained.

"I know," I responded. I tried to ignore it, but after a while I asked her to stop.

"If I could, do you think I'd be in this nuthouse?" she screamed.

After I knew her for a while, I got the feeling she was using her symptoms as a way to manipulate everyone around her. I talked to my supervisor about this and he recommended a game plan for my psychotherapy with her.

I asked Sarah about her earliest memory, a classic screening question in psychoanalysis.

"When I was a baby, I can remember my father yelling at my mother. And slapping her."

"Hmmm, yelling and slapping. Sound like anyone you know?" It's an easy interpretation, anyone could've seen it, but somehow, it still made an impression on her.

"You're good, Hollandaise."

If I Fell

I was still a resident at Mount Sinai in the spring of 1995, my third year of training, when I had the opportunity to plan an elective rotation. I opted for two months at Bellevue Hospital's psychiatric emergency room. As a visiting resident, I saw cases and reported directly to the attendings, working alongside the NYU residents. I told the Bellevue CPEP director that my residency schedule only allowed me to work Mondays, Wednesdays, and Fridays. I took off Tuesdays and Thursdays so I could have some time to myself to sleep in, do errands, and go running or Rollerblading. Some days I rode my bike through Central Park, my guitar slung over my shoulder, and played in Sheep's Meadow, a huge expanse of grass with a view of the midtown skyline. I needed this downtime between my frenetic days at the CPEP. The intensity of my experiences with the patients, crammed in with the other doctors in the tiny nurses' station, required a counterpoint. The trees rushing by me, the wind in my hair as I sped through the park, helped to recharge me. They were as essential for my mental health as the medications were for the patients, assuring that I remained a pod of sanity in a world of nuttery.

Monday, April 17, 1995. I had been at Bellevue for two weeks, and that night after work I was going to a party. My friend Dan Levy invited me to a gathering for Terence McKenna, the psychedelically inspired writer. I spent the bulk of my day with a new patient, a young man who came in floridly psychotic the night before. Luckily, I was able to track down his father in the Midwest who reported a history of bipolar disorder. My patient was off his meds and a long way from home. The CPEP was trying something new with these patients: high dose mood-stabilizers in an effort to bring them back to baseline more rapidly. I sat down with the patient to explain the treatment plan. He was funny, cute, and sweet, and we made a strong connection as the day wore on. I felt like he had a little bit of a crush on me, and I didn't do much to discourage him.

After my day at the ER, I changed into something that I hoped was fabulously sexy and headed downtown to the party. In a city full of numbered streets, I parked my car at the corner of White and Church, in front of the Baby Doll lounge. White and Church. Signs and omens. I wondered if I'd meet someone at the party, someone I would marry.

I walked from the corner to 395 Broadway, watching the litter swirl in the wind. I opened the door to the apartment. Cue the romantic music. Across a room filled with two dozen people, I saw a man who had seen me. I stared at him, thinking to myself, There he is, that's my guy: long, brown curly hair, beautiful blue-green eyes, full, sexy lips, strong chin. I had a strange feeling that he was The One I was supposed to be with. It felt preordained, inevitable; my only job was to accept it. It was irrational, but I was sure of it. The very definition of delusional.

I got up the courage to say something as I passed him on the way to the bathroom.

"Hi!" I said, in a tone that implied an old friendship, as if we already knew each other and I was glad to see him again.

"Hi?" He stared at me quizzically, in a tone that implied, *Do I know you?*

I hurried into the bathroom and leaned against the door as my heart pounded. *Pull yourself together, girl.* I waited a few minutes for my racing pulse and breathing to normalize, and left the bathroom.

I spent the rest of the evening chatting up every single person at the party, bar none. I shared a joint with Terence, then had a great stoned conversation with a brilliant young author, Doug Rushkoff, as I distractedly admired a young woman's behind, perfectly round and pert, unlike my own. But at all times, I always sensed exactly where He was in the room.

After the party, a group of us made plans to head down to Chinatown for dinner. As we gathered in the street, waiting for everyone to assemble, I asked Dan Levy to introduce me to Him. "This is Jeremy, my esteemed colleague," he said, and He and I chatted a bit as we walked to the restaurant. I arranged it so that Jeremy and I were seated together, and further, I separated him from the girl with the nice butt. I rubbed my leg against his. I flirted shamelessly, as did he. We began to speak to each other exclusively, as if no one else was around us. When I dared to look right at him, face-to-face, the Cher song in my head became deafening. "Take me home, take me home."

After drinks at a neighborhood bar, we walked back to his place, a fifth floor walk-up in Little Italy. The apartment was a classic cold-water flat, with the bathtub in the kitchen. I leaned against it as we kissed. Freedy Johnston's "Can You Fly" was playing in the background. The music, his kisses . . . it was all perfect.

"Well, good night," he teased, but I wasn't going anywhere and we both knew it.

In the morning, after a diner breakfast, he walked me to the corner of White and Church, and we leaned on my car as we kissed good-bye. When I got home, he had already emailed me his phone number. We talked on the phone for the better part of that night.

The next morning I went back into Bellevue, but it was as if I had been away for a year, I was so changed. I was in a parallel universe, orbiting around my new sun, obsessing grandiosely about our impending life together.

The manic patient I admitted to CPEP on Monday was still there. I was disappointed to see he was still quite disorganized, despite the heroic doses of mood-stabilizer he'd received, which had left him a bit unsteady on his feet but seemed to have had no other effect. He remembered me from two days before, though, and flashed me a huge grin, seeming awfully glad to see me again.

"How are you feeling, pally? Any better?" I asked him.

He was watching the TV in the ER waiting room. The Oklahoma bombing had just occurred, and the television coverage was exhaustive. He looked up at me, beaming. "I've been hit by the love bomb," he said proudly.

"Me too!" I replied.

Welcome to the Machine

After my Bellevue elective ended, I went back to Mount Sinai to finish my residency, and I continued to date Jeremy, the artist, photographer, writer, and my best boyfriend ever. Soon it was my fourth and final year, and I needed to decide what to do next. I applied for a schizophrenia research fellowship at Columbia and was accepted. I would be doing neuroimaging studies, analyzing PET scans of schizophrenics to try to discern the status of their serotonin receptors. I had been involved in schizophrenia research for most of my residency, had won an award from the National Institute of Mental Health for my protocol, and it was my assumption that this was my calling, my life's work. I was on the path I was meant to tread.

And then I got a phone call from Bellevue. Dr. Lear, the CPEP director, was offering me a job. "You made quite an impression when you rotated through here. We'd love to have you aboard."

I was flattered, to say the least. I hadn't applied for the job; they were calling me.

"So, here's the thing, Julie. It's not your typical schedule. We just need you to work weekends. Two overnights, Saturday and Sunday. And you'd need to come in for a few hours on Thursday mornings for faculty meetings."

"Just weekends?" I asked, incredulous. It was too good to be true. I could have all week off. To do what? Hang out with Jeremy and play guitar in the park? Take up ballet? Pottery? My mind was racing with the possibilities. It was more free time than I'd had in years, probably since summer vacations when I was a kid. And Bellevue was offering me significantly more money than Columbia. "But I already told Columbia I'd take the fellowship," I told him.

"Call them back and tell them you've changed your mind," he said casually, like this kind of thing happened all the time. "I need to know soon."

When I called Columbia to discuss it with the fellowship director, he was stupefied. No one had ever turned down a research fellowship at Columbia, it seemed.

I agonized over the decision for a few days, and drove Jeremy insane in the process. Even Dan Levy called it a "No-brainer! More money and more free time ... what's the dilemma exactly?" I seriously weighed taking both jobs and working seven days a week. Finally, I called the Columbia director back and sheepishly left a message on his machine, thanking him for all his help, but letting him know that I was taking the Bellevue job.

Two of Us

It is Monday, July 1, 1996, when I walk into the faculty offices of CPEP. Dr. Lear, my new boss, introduces me to some of the other doctors. And lo and behold, there is Lucy. I had actually forgotten all about her in the seven years since I'd brought her those wontons, but as soon as I hear her name and see her face, it all comes rushing back: the shirts, the stories, her balls, my blunder. ("Do your parents know?")

"And so we meet again!" I greet her. I wish that she would remember me immediately, but I have to mention the *mondu* before she does. I am thrilled to know we will be working together, and eager to attempt, once again, to befriend her.

I take Lucy as the ultimate good omen. If she likes it here, I know I will too. I idolized her at Temple, resonating with her energy so similar to my own. She was my doppelgänger, six years ahead of me in our training, but now our vectors have merged, and we are on the same playing field, both CPEP attendings. No longer an awed medical student and a strutting chief resident, we are now colleagues.

Now I know I'm in the right place.

Over the next few weeks, Lucy and I become fast friends at CPEP. As I get to know her better, she again lets me into her private inner sanctum, as she did that night in the Temple ER.

"Make sure you have good disability insurance," she says to me one day, pretty much out of the blue. "Get it now while you're young and healthy, and don't let it lapse."

"What are you talking about?" I ask.

"I'm going to let you in on a little something I haven't told everyone here. At my last job, before Bellevue, I had breast cancer. Radical mastectomy, chemo, radiation, the whole nine. I was thirty-one." We are standing in line at the coffee shop, getting breakfast. She tells me how incredibly sick she got, how even now anything orange, the color of the chemotherapy meds in the IV bag, can make her gag. How her white blood cell count got so low, her fevers so high, her oncologist didn't think she was going to pull through, but she did.

As if she weren't enough of a mythic figure in my eyes, Lucy Jones has beaten cancer. I call her accountant and get the pricey disability insurance.

Our faculty meetings are a smaller version of the weekly staff meetings: just the attending physicians are included. We meet on Thursday mornings after Lucy's overnight shift. She is giddy from lack of sleep and even more disinhibited than usual. It's my favorite time to be with her. She is wearing scrubs and is usually in need of a shower. There are times when I lean into her, seeing if her scent does anything for me, the way Jeremy's does. I love his smell; I can feel something stir in my pelvis when I breathe it in. I stare at her armpit hair, transfixed as it peeks out from her tank top. She doesn't shave there, like I do, like a man doesn't. She smiles at me and I blush. She has caught me, I think, but she lets it go. I am experimenting with an idea here, and I appreciate the latitude. We huddle in the corner, whispering and cracking wise. Dr. Lear has to separate us during the meetings as if we were schoolgirls. On Monday mornings, when I come in for rounds, I often say, "Good morning, Dr. Jones. . . . Good morning, everyone else." I do, on some level, separate her (or maybe it's us?) out from the rest. She rises easily above and beyond the other staff members, the cream above the crop. And I'm not the only one who places her on a pedestal. There are many of us at CPEP who speak of Lucy in blatantly worshipful language. She has a large group of idolizers, but the thing that I love best, that makes me feel special, is that she also admires me.

"Julie, sometimes I lie awake at night afraid you're smarter than I am," she says to me one morning. She smiles, and I know she's teasing me, but not totally. There is truth in her jest, and I lap it up like milk in a saucer. Soon we are a team, a mutual admiration society, and partners in crime.

We double-date with Sadie, her girlfriend, and Jeremy, inviting each other over for dinner to our apartments, or going down to Chinatown for Vietnamese food. Lucy and Sadie eventually buy a house together in the Hamptons, and they go there on the weekends. Jeremy and I can't hang out with them since that's when I work, but they generously offer us the use of the house during the week. The light in the late summer afternoons is like nothing I've ever seen. We go biking, windsurfing, kayaking. We eat lobsters and corn. We break their hammock with our combined weight, and I replace it, owning up to it when I see Lucy on Monday morning.

In the Bellevue of the Beast

I thought I knew what crazy was. Then I came to Bellevue.

I had already seen plenty of insanity, insinuating myself among the sickest psychiatric patients whenever possible during my eight years of training. I'd interviewed a guy at Temple who was hearing the Devil's voice while smelling burning flesh and seeing the flames of hell; I'd talked to a man at Mount Sinai with tinfoil under his hat to deflect the messages sent by the aliens; at the VA, I'd convinced a Vietnam veteran wearing a dead rat around his neck that we had better ways to protect him from his enemies.

These patients and their symptoms all pale in comparison to the pathology that parades through Bellevue's doors. The depth and breadth of madness on display at CPEP is like nothing I've ever experienced, and because of that, going to work is fascinating, illuminating, and exhilarating, week after week.

It's not until I start working at Bellevue that I finally appreciate what sets psychiatry apart from the rest of medicine. Medical illness has an endpoint: death. Psychosis is boundless; the degree to which someone can lose their mind is infinite. Most nights at CPEP, I'll think I've just seen the craziest patient ever, and then inevitably, a week later, a new patient will best the last.

Walking into my workplace is a bit like taking a hit of acid. I know all kinds of weird shit is going to go down, and I steel myself to handle it, because I also know that fifteen hours later I'm going to walk out the "other side." I just have to hold on tight and trust that it'll end with me still in one piece. One night I arrive at CPEP, and two patients in the observation area are both sweating and grunting. We have not one, but two women who believe they are giving birth. One of them swears it is the baby Jesus who will soon be delivered unto us. Those are the good nights, when the lunacy is funny, and going with the flow is painless. The nurses and psych techs (the staff in the nondetainable area, who have the most patient contact) strive to keep things light as we go about our business. All of us have chosen this line of work because we want to help others, but we learn over time that we have to set some limits. Most of us cauterize our bleeding hearts by using humor as a shield, so there is plenty of laughter erupting behind the scenes.

After just a few weekends at my new job, I see it's not going to be quite that easy. Treating everything as a joke will only get me so far. The problem is, I have a hair-trigger empathy switch, and because I am emotionally incontinent, my tear ducts leak with little provocation. If I see war, disasters, or orphans on the evening news or in the paper, my gut tightens and a lump forms in my throat. I can't abide the unfairness of it all. If I'm going to make it at CPEP, I have to find a way to tolerate hearing about the experiences of the mentally ill, the addicted, the unwanted. Maybe most people's lives are equal parts hope and despair, but at Bellevue, grief trumps optimism every time. There are sad stories everywhere. Pretty much every shift, if I let it get to me, there's at least one patient's story that will tear me up inside.

So I start to toughen up. I can't allow myself to get bogged down in the darkness, so I choose to have a little bit of a negative charge around me to keep it at bay. I adjust my filter a bit, tweaking the EQ so the sympathy frequency is turned way down. I pretend I don't care, and after a while, I start to believe it. I pretend nothing fazes me, and pretty soon, it seems like nothing does.

To prevent the misery from overwhelming me, I strip away the pitiful details and focus on the bottom line. Where does this patient need to go? Is he a keeper? Will he survive if I send him back out to the city streets? Or will someone else be in danger if I release him?

To the outside observer, I appear hardened, uncaring. Maybe other people would play it a different way, but this is my game plan. I am all business, except that I go for the cheap laugh whenever I can, whether with the ambulance drivers and cops or the Bellevue police, nurses, and psych techs. But on the inside, if you could hear my interior monologue, it is pure Kurtz . . . "The horror." I am aghast at the indignities these patients endure, and there are occasionally times I am afraid for my own safety.

I can laugh all I want, just like a teenager on acid, but I'm kidding myself if I think I'm going to walk out of here unchanged.

By the time I leave, nine years later, my suit of armor will have become dented and worn through with rust. A working mother of two with a heart of mush, I will be unable to harden myself any longer to the atrocities to which I bear witness.

I'd love to tell you that it was a gradual, step-by-step progression, from hard-ass to maternal, that it was a smooth narrative arc. I know that's how a good screenplay would read; but in truth, my growth came in fits and starts, and I had to learn the same lessons repeatedly before they'd sink in. One step forward, a couple back, a couple more forward: Eventually I inched my way along the path, growing and changing, but the process wasn't pretty.

To Protect and Serve

I usually start off my Saturday night shifts by cleaning up the trash, throwing away all the used coffee cups, pen caps, and progress notes. Once the area seems a bit neater, I get to work on "clearing the rack." Tonight, there is a backlog of patients who have been seen and put on Hold. This means the doctor on the shift before mine couldn't make up his mind about what to do with them, or else the patients were too drunk or high to be released. Most Holds get discharged once they're sober (they've "cleared" in medical terms), but other times we admit them to a detox bed, or, if they look psychiatrically sick enough, to the dual diagnosis ward upstairs for the MICA patients—mentally ill, chemical-abusing—an acronym that efficiently describes most of our patients.

I grab the first chart from the Hold bin: a guy who was wandering the hospital's hallways last night, high on cocaine. When HP tried to escort him out, he made only enough sense to convey that he felt suicidal. Now, nearly twenty-four hours later, he says he feels better; he's come down off his high and is eager to put his Bellevue detour behind him. That makes two of us, but he won't let me call anyone to confirm that he isn't a suicide risk or an axe-murderer.

"Mr. DiCarlo, I can't let you go until I can speak with someone who can vouch for you. I need a phone number of a friend, a cousin . . . anyone."

He sits and stews for a while, not willing to give up a number. After a couple of hours of waiting, he realizes I'm not kidding. The number is his only ticket out.

"Okay. You can call my mother, but she doesn't speak much English."

I approximate Italian using my meager Spanish, and she manages to communicate two things to me:

1) Don't send him here.
2) He beats his girlfriend.

She gives me the girlfriend's phone number slowly in her native tongue.

I know I have to call the girlfriend. Somehow, I sense I can't release him unless she gives the go-ahead. He's in a hurry to get discharged and is pressuring me to let him go, and if there's one thing I've learned in my few months at CPEP it's this: If they want to stay, they need to leave; if they want to leave, they need to stay. It seems to hold true ninety-five percent of the time. If someone walks in saying, "I am hearing voices telling me to kill myself and others," or "I am a danger to myself and others," then I know he is relaying verbatim what he's learned on the street, in the shelters, or in jail. He believes this will get him "three hots and a cot" in the hospital for a few days. If a patient is trying his hardest to be released, but won't give up any phone numbers that can make it happen, then I have to assume something is amiss.

"Mr. DiCarlo, I need to talk to your girlfriend."

"I want out of here," he grimaces. "I'm done with your phone calls."

"You cannot leave here until I talk to your girlfriend."

"That isn't going to happen."

He doesn't know I have her phone number already. "Fine," I reply. "You can rot here all weekend for all I care." I'm being a bully, and for some reason, he is eating it up. He doesn't bolt for the door, he doesn't escalate to the point of being restrained. He wants the conflict to be drawn out.

Eventually I get in touch with his girlfriend and ask her if she will feel safe if he is discharged.

"Don't let him out!" she begs me.

She tells me she has an order of protection against him which he's violated continually for the past two weeks, and the police are looking for him. Two weeks ago, he busted down her door, pulled the phone out of the wall while she was trying to call the cops, beat her up, and choked her until she was blue, all the while telling her that he was going to kill her because he loved her. She explains how all of this happened because she went out with some other guy and told my patient they were through. Her father had to pull him off of her and hold him down until the police came and arrested him. He was eventually released from custody, and by then she had gotten the order of protection. She thinks this will protect her, but here's another thing I've learned at Bellevue: An order of protection does not actually protect you. It's a court order, not a magical shield around your apartment. (I always abbreviate it as OOPs! when I take notes during a sign-out.)

She goes on to explain that he's been harassing her by phone and threatening her life every time he contacts her, so . . . no, she does not feel safe if he is discharged. As a matter of fact, he's been calling her from our ER, telling her that he's on his way over there to finish the job as soon as he's released.

I document his exact words in the chart: "You're dead. You are dead when I get there, do you hear me? I am coming over there to kill you. I don't care: I'll do the twenty-five to life."

Honestly, I marvel at this guy's balls. He's in a hospital ER, talking on the patient phone in a public area, steps away from the hospital policeman sitting at his desk, and he's threatening his ex-girlfriend's life. The HP on tonight, Rocky, is collapsed in the corner as usual, reading his body-building magazine, oblivious. I call the local police precinct and explain the situation, and they ask me to detain the patient until they can arrive. It is a felony to violate an order of protection.

I call the girlfriend back and let her know that the patient will be locked up, first at Bellevue in our ER, and then downtown at central booking, so she is safe for now. She is crying and thanking me and telling me I have saved her life, which is very sweet. And possibly true.

I sit at the desk in the nurses' station for a moment, feeling relieved that this story will have a happy ending, sort of. (There's no white knight and swooning princess, but at least no one gets killed.) I came pretty close to discharging this guy without calling anyone. He was initially held because he told someone he was suicidal. Once the drugs left his system, he denied suicidal ideation, and typically that would be enough to get the ball rolling on a discharge.

The thing is . . . it isn't just the issue of danger to self, it is also the possibility of danger to others that allows me—and compels me, even as I'm trying to "clean up the area"—to retain a patient against his will. I need to cover all the bases. He denies suicidality, fine, but what else? If I had let this guy go, I have no doubt he would have gone back over to her apartment and killed his girlfriend, or attempted to. And it would have been because I thought he was fine to leave, and was in too much of a hurry to bother with due diligence.

I go into the holding area to tell the patient that the police are coming to get him.

"How can you believe her over me?" he whines. "I just love her so much."

To which I reply, "You've got a funny way of showing your love, pal." I spin around, thus ending our conversation with a bit of dramatic flair. I am a couple of steps away from the nurses' station when I hear a WHUMP!

I turn to see Chuck, the large male nurse who is a dead ringer for Kenny Rogers. He is kneeling on the floor with his elbow poised over Mr. DiCarlo's Adam's apple.

"I told you I had a bad feeling about this guy," Chuck grunts. Seeing the patient following me into the doorway of the nurses' station and assuming he was about to attack me, Chuck put his arm around the guy's torso and flipped him onto the ground quick as a flash.

"Chuck, you are my hero, ya big tattooed thug!" I squeal. He is the closest thing I have to a big brother in the ER; his protective stance helps to reinforce the feelings of family that pervade my shifts at the hospital. Chuck has my back, literally. Rocky, on the other hand, is nowhere to be seen.

A few weeks later, I call the girlfriend to make sure she is okay, still safe, maybe getting some counseling, and . . . you guessed it. She's back with our bad boy.

I hang up the phone feeling exactly the way I used to when I worked at Filene's Basement. I'd spend an hour meticulously folding a bin full of tangled button-down shirts, only to come back later in my shift to find the bin as sloppy as it was when I started, all because someone was searching for a seventeen-inch neck. It was like I'd never been there, organizing the mess. Like I hadn't done my job.

I remember learning about entropy in college physics class: The natural order of things is disorder. Chaos reigns supreme throughout the universe, especially at Bellevue. I can't beat it, so I may as well join it.

Most important, I learn not to call patients for follow-up. I'd rather pretend the shirts remain neatly folded and organized.

I'm Looking Through You

Psychiatrists don't typically use stethoscopes and tongue depressors, conducting a physical exam the way other doctors do. We don't need to lay a hand on our patients to make a diagnosis. We perform a mental status exam, a noninvasive way of seeing how the patient's mind is functioning.

Some of the mental status exam can be done from across the room, for instance evaluating appearance and behavior. Being an ER shrink means that I am allowed to judge a book by its cover. I can unabashedly make conclusions about someone's mood based on their fashion sense, for instance. In a manic state, with excessive energy and inflated self-esteem, a patient may be wearing bright, clashing colors, garish makeup, or an elaborate Carmen Miranda headdress. (I have a saying at CPEP: "Headdress equals mania until proven otherwise.") Manic patients tend to over-groom, sometimes shaving their bodies or plucking out all their eyebrows, other times overdoing lipstick and liner, straying far beyond the lip's natural contour.

Conversely, depressed patients may under-groom. Their clothes are disheveled and dirty, their hair may be greasy or in need of a new dye-job. Fingernails are the windows into the soul, if you ask me. I always make a point of checking nails and cuticles, looking for outward manifestations of internal anxiety states. These are signs of what could be considered "neurotic self-mutilation." Many patients called "cutters" have arrays of symmetrical cuts on their arms, for example. Psychotic self-mutilation is more extreme and dangerous: I remember a woman at Temple who'd tried to give herself a homemade Cesarean when she heard her unborn baby crying to be let out. As I chat with a patient, I try to look surreptitiously for scars on wrists, alerting me to past suicide attempts, or track-marks on arms, betraying a history of intravenous drug abuse. Although New York City is full of people who have pierced and tattooed themselves beyond recognition, I still take note. Tattoos on the face and neck in particular get my attention, warning me I may be dealing with an antisocial personality.

Another thing I need to gauge is a patient's psychomotor activity. If he is pacing, fidgeting, or wringing his hands, it will be documented in the chart that he is psychomotor agitated. Conversely, when someone reaches a significant level of depression, his movements can become labored and sluggish, called psychomotor retardation. If a patient is paranoid, he may appear hyper-vigilant, repeatedly looking over his shoulders, or he may place his back to the wall, unwilling to have anyone stand behind him.

I pride myself on intuiting what drugs a patient took just by looking at him. Someone who is strung out on speed (methamphetamine) is typically wiry, jumpy, pale, and thin. Sweaty black concert T-shirts, acne, and tribal tattoos are the norm. Crack intoxication is all about twitching, jawing, and grimacing. These movements are called dyskinesias and are the result of too much dopamine flooding the brain. Someone who is high on opiates (heroin, methadone, or prescription painkillers like Oxycontin) has an ultrarelaxed face with slack cheek muscles, the eyes at half-mast. It is called "on the nod" because the head, often with a pleasant half-smile, will jerk up after the chin dips down to the chest.

Pupils are important to pay attention to; I'm always reminding the residents who work with me, "The pupils don't lie." They will dilate under the influence of many drugs that act as stimulants, like cocaine, speed, and hallucinogens. If someone comes into CPEP high on opiates the pupils will be constricted to pinpoints. Because all drugs derived from the poppy can slow down the respiratory rate, I need to count breaths per minute. Any fewer than ten and the patient needs to be quickly shuttled to the medical ER to be treated for an overdose with an opioid antagonist called Narcan.

Once I've given a patient the visual once-over, the rest of the mental status exam involves having a conversation. Initially, I need to assess his level of attention and concentration. I'll ask, "What's your name? Do you know where you are? Can you tell me what day it is?" while I'm also ascertaining if he's intoxicated, sedated, stimulated, or distracted. If a patient is alert, or even hyper-alert, I can proceed with the interview, but many times at Bellevue patients are simply too drunk or high to have a meaningful conversation, and I need to let them sleep it off on a stretcher before I can do a good exam.

Typically, I start with questions that won't be considered too invasive or personal. Orienting questions like "Where are we now? What's the name of this place?" establish if the patient is firmly rooted in the here and now, and are an easy way to break the ice. They help set the tone for the rest of the interview as well, reminding the patient that I am a psychiatrist and this won't be a normal, everyday conversation.

It is crucial for me to make sure the patient is medically stable as early as possible, so I ask questions about current medications, drug allergies, and a history of medical illness. Some acute medical conditions can masquerade as psychiatric ones, and the consequences can be deadly if I miss this. I may also ask, "Are you supposed to be taking any medicines you've decided not to take?" Plenty of people come to Bellevue off of their lithium or antipsychotics, and this is a useful piece of data to gather early in the game.

At the top of the page of the CAF, the Comprehensive Assessment Form which gets filled out on every patient, I must document my own evaluation of the patient's reliability. Some people are genuine, accurately reporting symptoms and psychiatric histories. Others are ingratiating, evasive, seductive, or hostile. This can tell me a tremendous amount about personality structure, and also what the level of motivation is for seeking treatment or avoiding it. Many have ulterior motives: the patient who wants to be certified as disabled, the abandoned girlfriend who wants her boyfriend to feel guilty, the prisoner who is looking for a hospital bed instead of a jail cell. Mostly, when there's only one informant, I need to rely on my gut to tell me who's lying. Sometimes friends, family members, employers, therapists, or probation officers (called collateral contacts) can give me a fuller picture, helping to confirm or refute what the patient is reporting. Occasionally I'll find myself in the midst of a "he said/she said" situation, but usually it's easy enough to tease apart the reality from the added layers of lies and drama.

Funny thing, being a psychiatrist, you'd think I'd be used to drama, to the gnashing and wailing of people in distress, but I'm not. Actually, I can't stand it. Genuine emotion is one thing. I know it when I see it and I can ease my way around it, working to get to the information I need to make a diagnosis and make a difference. It's the blatantly manufactured melodrama that nauseates me. But I let that work in my favor. If I'm not feeling sympathetic, chances are it's my sixth sense telling me I shouldn't be.

A taxi driver once asked me what I did for a living. "I'm a psychiatrist," I answered warily.

"Oho! So . . . you know what I'm thinking right now?" he asked. He wasn't joking. He honestly thought that I was a mind reader. People sometimes clam up when they find out I'm a shrink, afraid I'll be able to peer into their souls and know their darkest secrets. I wish it were that easy. Once people start to open up, I begin to see where their issues are, but if they don't talk, I can't possibly know what's going on in their minds. Psychiatry isn't neurosurgery. We have no trick for getting inside someone's head. You speak, we analyze. You don't talk, we got nuthin'.

Scrutinizing a patient's speech and its structure is crucial to establishing the diagnosis. Answers can be concise and goal-directed, or the words can wander off in various directions. In mania, the speech is pressured, tongue-twistingly fast and difficult to interrupt. The patient will suddenly shift gears, moving from one topic to the next. If I pay close attention to this "flight of ideas," I can usually see a thread linking the topics, and it is often poetic in its beauty. Schizophrenics can have disorganized speech, a reflection of disordered thoughts. Either the patient will go off on a tangent and never return, or the speech is so muddled it stops making sense and is referred to as "word salad."

There is a form of psychosis called catatonia that is so severe, the brain seems to shut down the speech centers entirely. It's not just the mouth that is paralyzed; the rest of the muscles of the body behave strangely as well. If I move a patient's limb, it will stay in its new spot, no matter how gravity-defying. This is called waxy flexibility. The first time I met a catatonic schizophrenic, I walked into the interview room, introduced myself, and extended my hand. He stared straight ahead, his frozen face expressionless. Lights on, nobody home. I initially thought the patient rude for not returning my greeting and shaking my hand! It wasn't until I checked for waxy flexibility that I realized what was going on.

In CPEP, I learned to allow patients to remain in a catatonic state for a while. As long as their blood pressure, and heart and respiratory rates, remain stable, it is better not to rush them into the next phase. But if necessary, it is usually not difficult to "break a catatonia." An injection of any member of the benzodiazepine family of medicines (like Valium or Ativan) will loosen up the muscles, the brain, and the mouth. The problem is, underneath that quiet exterior lurks a severe psychosis. Most catatonics break loud, so when the CPEP is noisy enough, the nurses and I typically agree that there's no reason to go upsetting the applecart. We won't rush to medicate someone who is mute because, more often than not, we still won't have any useful information once they start talking.

There are other times, however, when there is nothing more irritating, nor more challenging for me to handle, than a patient's silence. Catatonia is an involuntary mutism; the patient is physiologically unable to speak. A patient who remains mute voluntarily is another story. It is a simple thing to do, requiring a modest amount of persistence and will, but it is a cunning ploy and its effects are potent: The case cannot be closed if the patient will not participate in the interview. It's a great stalling tactic, frustrating as hell for the attending psychiatrist who is trying to keep things moving in a busy ER. When confronted with a prisoner who won't talk, I marvel at how easily I am thwarted and placed in a powerless position. It is genius in its simplicity. *I will surely do the same if I am ever arrested,* I think to myself. But I doubt I could pull it off. I am a huge talker. This is likely the reason why I find myself almost in awe of the mute patient. I'd have to be in a coma to keep quiet.

After gathering information on appearance, behavior, and speech, I need to delve deeper, appraising a patient's thoughts and perceptions. Sometimes it's obvious the patient is hearing voices. From my years as a medical student doing research on auditory hallucinations, I know how to recognize when I am speaking with people who are actively hallucinating. There are a few tip-offs to look for: They will dart their eyes or head toward the perceived source of the voices, and their speech will be fragmented. This is because if someone is speaking to you while you're speaking, it is impossible to be fluid in your speech. The brain cannot both listen to incoming words and create coherent conversation. (Have a friend whisper in your ear while you try to talk and you'll see.)

A crucial piece of information to extract during the mental status exam is whether the patient is suicidal. There is a continuum of suicidality: a spectrum that spans from having passive thoughts ("It'd just be easier if I didn't exist"), to suicidal fantasies ("I wish I were dead"), to intention ("I'm going to kill myself"). In the same way that it is customary to sneeze if you have a cold, it is common to have suicidal fantasies if you are depressed. Suicidal thoughts, especially if they feel foreign and upsetting to the patient, are less worrisome than specific plans, actions, or intent. If a patient has developed a blueprint for ending his life, if he has started to act on this plan and has the intention of carrying it out, it is obviously much more dangerous than someone who is simply musing about how all his troubles would go away if he were to go to sleep and never wake up.

Statistically, people who have a history of suicide attempts are more likely to try again. I don't beat around the bush when asking questions about suicidal thoughts and histories. A lot of people are relieved to finally share them with someone. In the CPEP, we err on the side of caution and keep a patient for observation or a short admission if there is any threat of suicide or self-harm.

The last part of the mental status exam is about insight and judgment. Does the patient think anything is wrong with him or that everything is fine? Does he accept recommendations for treatment, or is he chronically noncompliant? Schizophrenia is often characterized by poor insight into the presence of the illness, and patients in a manic state frequently make foolhardy decisions. In either case, this can accentuate the dangerousness of their situation. Impaired insight typically worsens a prognosis, and having poor judgment in New York City puts you at risk in a million different ways.

Psychiatrists assess judgment by asking standard questions, such as, "If you found a stamped, addressed letter, what would you do with it?" I prefer to get a gestalt from the patient's retelling of recent events. Someone who explains that he cut off his right hand because the Bible says to do so "if it offends thee," I can easily deem to have poor judgment. Ditto the man asking to be injected with Perrier to quiet his voices.

But then there are the cases that could go either way. My passing judgment on the quality of someone else's can be influenced by all sorts of information. One of my earliest patients at Bellevue was a man who asked me, "Do you think I'm nuts, or just bananas, because my brother is a total meatball!"

I told him, with a wink, "I doubt your diagnosis is nuts; I think it's overused, actually. However, I can't rule out bananas, or even partial meatball, but I haven't yet seen a case of total meatball. I'd like to meet your brother sometime."

The patient smiled at my response, which I took to be a good sign, but later he asked me to marry him. I didn't hold that against him, but I did admit him.

I Don't Want to Spoil the Party

It's my first Christmas at Bellevue, December 1996, and I volunteer to cover the CPEP. Ever since medical school, being a nice Jewish doctor, I've gone out of my way to volunteer to work Christmas Day, or Christmas Eve, or both. I have no family obligations, plus it's always fun to work holidays in the hospital, because people are in a good mood, there's lots of home-cooked food around, and sometimes a little spiked eggnog or tasty coquito when no one's looking. Working the holiday also gives me a chance to reminisce about my fourth year of medical school, the time I volunteered to work on Christmas because I knew I'd be paired up with the dreamy surgeon, and we ended up having sex in the call-room most of the day, because there were no surgeries booked.

On my regular weekends, I have to go upstairs to the inpatient wards and write notes on the new patients before I start my work in the ER. Responsibility for these notes is divided between me and one of the moonlighters—the doctors-for-hire who work in the CPEP and upstairs during the weekends and holidays. But on weekday holidays, the attending isn't supposed to leave the CPEP to go upstairs to write notes; the moonlighter must write all of them himself. Since I'm in charge of the CPEP today, it's my job to assign the up-wards note-writing to another doctor. I pick Martin, the up-wards moonlighter for the day.

I'm not looking forward to telling him the news. He hates taking orders from me, and we've clashed before on cases where I had to pull rank. He may be older than I am, and he may come from a culture where women are not usually in charge, but right now I am his boss and I have to give this task to one of my underlings.

"Hey, Martin . . . I'm sorry to tell you, but you've got some extra notes to do this afternoon." I take a deep breath to explain. "It's a holiday. I know that the attending does the up-wards notes on the weekends, but it's a weekday today, and it needs to be assigned to another doctor."

"But you're the weekend attending and you're here," he argues.

"On the weekends, I come in early to do the notes. It's Monday morning and I have to stay in the ER all day. I can't leave to go upstairs for that long. I need to assign a moonlighter to do it," I explain.

"I'm not going to do your work," he informs me.

"Martin, just write the notes. It's not that big a deal."

"It's not right," he complains. "I'm going to call Dr. Lear."

I am incredulous as he dials the phone. How he knows our boss's home number is beyond me, and I am flabbergasted that he thinks this is important enough to warrant disturbing him on Christmas Day.

I can hear Dr. Lear's voice through the receiver as he talks to Martin.

Dr. Lear is succinct and unambiguous: Dr. Holland is in charge. My colleague has no choice but to do what he is told. Only he doesn't.

When Dr. Lear comes back from Christmas vacation and learns that Martin's work was not done, he fires him from the moonlighting pool. I think nothing more about it. I've got bigger fish to fry.

The hospital police officer who is frequently assigned to the CPEP on the weekend nights always seems to be sleeping. If Rocky isn't leafing through his inevitable bodybuilding magazines or chatting me up, he's got his head craned back, his chin pointed to the ceiling and his mouth agape. Sometimes I stand in front of him while he snores to see how soundly he's asleep. Other times, I will startle him awake and give him a withering look. This guy is supposed to be protecting me so *I* can sleep! Dr. Lear has made it clear that the attendings can sleep overnight if the residents have things under control. But I don't feel very safe with my call-room down the hall from the detainable area if there's no one guarding the hallway.

I decide to write a letter to the head of the hospital police, complaining about Rocky.

A few weeks later, Chuck is attacked by a female patient who is trying to escape. She charges out the door, makes it to the clerk's desk and grabs a heavy black metal three-hole-punch. When Chuck chases her and attempts to get her to return to CPEP, she whacks him in the face with the three-hole-punch. Rocky wrestles her down and brings her back to her chair, dragging her in with another HP. Chuck ends up in the medical ER getting sutures across the bridge of his nose.

Several weeks after the attack, I am summoned to a meeting involving Rocky. I assume it is about the letter I wrote. I walk cautiously into a room reserved for the hospital police, on the other side of the hospital. Rocky is sitting behind a desk, his wide chest wrapped in a suit and tie, flanked by a union representative. I am nervous that I'm getting him fired. I just wanted his boss to tell him not to sleep on the job. A simple reprimand. Why is this office set up like a courtroom? I am asked to approach the table and state my name. There is someone acting like a judge, a mediator I assume. I feel like I've been shanghaied.

"Doctor Holland, can you tell us what happened on the night when Chuck, the nurse on duty, was attacked?" asks the mediator.

"W-well," I stammer, licking my lips. This is about Chuck? "I was sleeping at the time of the incident, so I could only tell you what I've heard."

"Can you tell me if you witnessed this hospital police officer assaulting a patient?" the mediator asks as he points at Rocky.

"What?" I yelp. "Assaulting who?"

"The patient who allegedly assaulted the nurse on duty, did you see any altercation between her and any hospital police officer?"

"No. I didn't see anything. I was sleeping." Rocky smiles at me, thanking me with his eyes. What the hell is going on? What did he do? "Excuse me, but can you tell me what this is about? Is Rocky being accused of something?"

"Yes, ma'am. The patient states that he kicked her in the leg."

This seems like a pretty formal inquisition for one kick in the leg. "This has nothing to do with the letter I wrote? Complaining about him sleeping at his post?" I ask. I want his union rep to know that I'm not the best person to call in as a character witness in his case. But it's too late. Rocky is looking relieved, like they don't have any proof of whatever it is he did if I don't condemn him.

I suppose it's better if Rocky thinks I've helped him instead of focusing on my letter. I already got Martin fired; I don't want to get anyone else pissed off at me. Rocky and I will be working together for years to come, and I need him to watch my back. Fortunately, we will be relocating the CPEP to a new wing of the hospital in a few months. The call-rooms will be across the hall in a separate locked area. I won't care if Rocky is sleeping while I am, as long as there are two locked doors separating me from the detainable area.

Mama Told Me Not to Come

Sunday night in late fall, it's Chuck's birthday, and also the eve of mine. We begin a tradition of celebrating our birthdays together when we work the same weekend. I have made a fudge-marble layer cake with mocha frosting. (The secret ingredient is an extra packet of vanilla pudding added to the cake mix.) We light the candles around midnight, each singing to the other, surrounded by nurses and psych techs. We stand on either side of the cake as we hold the plate, blowing the candles out when our song ends.

Our singing is halfhearted, and we certainly can't compare with the crooning female patient EMS has just brought in, wrapped in a body bag. The NYC body bags are made of canvas and mesh; they are navy blue, and look like fashionable, oversized totes. These Velcro devices quickly turn an agitated and unmanageable person into a piece of luggage. When the patient is horizontal and wrapped up in the bag, there are sturdy straps that make it easier to heave him onto a stretcher. There is a peroxide-blond woman sitting in the nondetainable area and I assume she is a patient waiting to be seen, but I soon discover that she is one of the EMS workers. Along with two cops and her partner, she parades the new patient over to the triage nurse. The patient in the body bag is a woman in her thirties with long, curly hair and a strident voice. She is singing various songs at the top of her lungs, the best of which is "Mama Told Me Not to Come" by Three Dog Night. She doesn't want to be here; her mama said there'd be days like this.

She calls everyone "babe," in a casual, yet demeaning tone. It's her way of equalizing the power structure, I figure. She is naked and immobilized in the blue canvas restraint, amid a room full of people in uniforms. I'd be calling everybody "babe," too.

"What's with the body burrito?" I ask the cop.

His eyes crinkle at my joke as the EMS driver steps in to give me the rundown. "Her landlord called 911 after her tub overfilled and damaged the apartment below hers. He also said she was blasting her music and that she was naked out on the fire escape." It's frigid outside, so I have to factor that in. The driver continues, "When the cops came, she started singing the lyrics to the Stevie Nicks album she was listening to, and jumped into and out of the tub. Then she pulled out a pipe and attempted to smoke something in front of the police, offering to share."

The blond EMS driver jokes with me about how she's as crazy as the patients, as I nod and smile nervously back at her. She tells me that before she worked for EMS, she used to be a belly dancer who once garnered an offer of a million dollars from some visiting Saudis to dance for them privately. She turned them down.

"Is that the crazy part?" I ask.

Whenever I try to talk to my new patient, explaining where she is and what will happen next, she sings so loudly that I can't get a word in edgewise. I finally give up and write the medication orders for sedation, filling out the paperwork for a 9.39. There is a lull afterwards, and I start to gather up my belongings to head to my office when two New York City policemen roll in an arrested man, who is yelling, "You got the wrong guy!" repeatedly.

"You guys unloaded?" I ask the cops. It's practically my standard greeting with NYPD. They have to unload their weapons before entering CPEP. I wonder if they resent the hospital policy. Maybe it's uncomfortable for them to be carrying useless guns. Maybe it's even more awkward when I confront them with their impotence; it somehow calls their manhood into question.

"Yes, ma'am," they both reply.

"What'd you bring me?" I ask the younger-looking one.

"Male black, twenty-nine, arrested for drug possession with intent to distribute." The cops always talk backwards, Male Black, Female Hispanic. No one else presents cases this way. "When he got arraigned, he started screaming, telling off the judge, and then he went back into his cell and trashed the place. The judge wants him here." The cop grins. "We shouldn't get all the fun, right?"

"They sent him to Bellevue as if there's something psychiatrically wrong with this guy? He's just acting up, right? Is he saying anything crazy?"

"Not crazy, but he's pretty threatening."

The prisoner taunts the police, his chin jutted out while he howls, "I . . . HAVE . . . A . . . RAZOR! It's hidden on me. You're never gonna find it. I'll pull it out later and cut all your faces."

As he is being searched, his pockets emptied one by one, he shrieks at the police, "It's not in my pants! Don't cut my pants! I hid it up my ass! I'm gonna pull it out later and I will fuck you up. I swear on my dead mother that I'll do it."

"Chuck, we need to five and four this guy," I say, meaning 5 mg of Haldol and 4 mg of Ativan. Two fairly large doses, but I'm guessing that's what we'll need to put him down. It takes every staff member we have, all the NYPD cops and all the hospital police in the area to hold the patient down while Chuck injects the medication into his gluteus muscle. He could've just injected it into his arm, but I'm thinking, *Maybe he feels like playing hardball?* It's his birthday, too, so I let it go.

The patient is boiling mad now. "I'm gonna fuck you up with that razor, just like you fucked me up with that needle. I'm gonna cut all o' you . . . fuck you up good."

"Sir, if you keep telling us you have a razor hidden inside you, we're going to have to search you there as well," I say, balancing sounding polite with seeming menacing.

"I'm gonna sue the hospital. You can't Abner Louima me! My family's gonna sue your asses," he threatens.

I look to Chuck, who motions with his head toward the guy. "I guess you gotta check him, Doc."

I've done rectal exams aplenty in medical school. If he needs to be checked, I certainly know how to do it. "Okay, you guys, anybody here do yoga? You know the plow position?" The cops look at me quizzically, and I explain what we're going to do. "Flip his legs up over his head so I can get to his ass."

The patient becomes silent and passive, for reasons I can't begin to imagine, as we guide his legs, his pants around his ankles, up over his head. I put on a pair of gloves and opt to do without the Surgilube, which typically would help to lubricate a gloved finger into the rectum on a normal exam. I have no idea if there's any lube in the CPEP, and I don't have time to go hunting it down.

But it's more than that. I'm surrounded by six tough guys, and I'm trying to act like one too, getting caught up in their game. I might as well be grabbing my crotch, swearing, spitting, and talking about sports. The posturing that men do, the armor that they wear . . . they do it to protect their hearts, and their balls. With their phallic guns, bullets, and missiles, they aim to be the penetrators, not the penetrated. Stupidly, I want to be like them. I slip into my butch mode so I can fit in.

As my finger pushes haltingly inside his warm body, it occurs to me that if he does have a razor up his ass, I could well get my finger sliced.

"No razor," I tell Chuck, relieved. I turn to the cops and say flippantly, "He's clean, so to speak." I strip the glove off, flipping it inside out with a snap, and walk into the nurses' station.

"He's got no psych history, he doesn't appear psychotic, and he's not disorganized. We'll put him on Hold and send him back to NYPD when he calms down a little," I say to my imaginary audience as I grab his chart off the rack.

I am at home the next day when Lucy calls me. "Hey, Jules. You know that prisoner you put on Hold last night? Right after morning rounds, they found a razor on his stretcher by his head. He was sleeping, so they just tossed it, but he really could've cut somebody up."

"Are you sure?" I ask. "I searched him, Lucy! He was telling everyone how he had a razor hidden up his ass. I personally stuck my finger up that guy's butt. There was no razor."

"Are you nuts? What did you do that for? Jesus, Julie, what if he did have a razor up his ass? You could've cut your finger to bits!"

I can't explain it, of course. What came over me? Why stoop to his level? Why be so sadistic? But I expect Lucy, of all people, to understand me. Her immediate reaction lets me know that I've stepped over the line. I am shamed, and worst of all, he clearly did have a razor hidden somewhere, and I missed it. Where the hell was it?

"I don't know what to tell you, Luce. I guess this place is just getting to me or something."

"Julie," she says in her charming Southern accent, "I'll tell you what I'm going to do. I'm going to consult our friendly CPEP Bible on this one. We'll let the good word of the Lord tell us how you should've handled this guy." She opens the copy of the New Testament which has been hanging around the bookshelf in the nurses' station for the past few weeks.

"I've been using the New Testament like the *I Ching* recently, and it hasn't let me down yet. I'm going to pick a random verse from the book, and that will give us holy, divine guidance on what to do with this sort of patient. Okay, here we go." She reads the verse into the phone:

"Away with such a fellow from the earth, for he is
not fit to live."
Acts 22, Chapter 22, Verse 22

"Well! I guess now we have our answer," she hoots.

I am amazed. The Bible. Yet there's no "Turn the other cheek," no "Love thy neighbor as thyself."

"All right, then," I say. "I guess that's that."

"Yep. That is that."

"But Luce, seriously. Think about what I did."

"Don't worry about it, baby. We all go there at some point. Well, you and I go there, anyway. Remember the time I totally attacked that patient who was being a dick to everybody? And how Chuck had to pull me off him?"

"How can I forget?" I say. "Between you and Chuck, I've heard about it enough times." I'm probably a little jealous: When Chuck tells how Lucy manhandled the guy, his eyes mist over at the memory. Instead of proving our manhood to our fathers, now Lucy and I are unconsciously using Chuck to judge the competition. Lucy is winning. "Anyway, I'm sorry about the razor. I truly have no idea how it got by me."

"No harm, no foul, right?" says Lucy.

"Right. No one was hurt. You letting that guy go or what?"

"It's already taken care of," she chirps. "He is O.T.D."

Out the door. Good. "Back to the cops?" I ask, though I know the answer. He's an arrested prisoner. There's nowhere else he could go.

It's just that I don't want to hang up the phone yet. I always love talking to Lucy. Her down-home drawl envelops me, like a mint-julep blanket.

"Hell yeah! You think I'm gonna let the razor man back onto the street?" she crows. "Hey, Julie."

"Yeah?"

"Happy birthday, girl."

"Thanks, pal."

The Wind Cries Mary

After our Thursday morning faculty meeting, I'm hanging out with Lucy in her call-room down the hall from the CPEP. In her cramped office is a small bed beside a chair and desk, a telephone and reading lamp on its edge.

I need to talk with her about what happened with the razor man. I'm worried about my level of sadism, how quickly I can transform from Dorothy to the Wicked Witch.

"I went through the same thing when I first got here. Eventually it settles down, you find your pacing. Talking about it helps. I've got a great shrink for you if you want. I know she's got an opening 'cause I just wrapped up with her." She writes the number of her therapist down for me on a rectangular Post-it note, emblazoned with the name of a new antipsychotic drug, courtesy of one of the many visiting drug reps.

My new therapist's name, written in Lucy's commanding capital letters, is Mary Shears. Lucy is handing me a savior named Mary. Mother of God. That's gotta be a good sign, right? From a psychotherapeutic point of view, it will be easier for me to have the corrective emotional experience of a caring and articulate mother if she's got the ultimate maternal name. The Shears part triggers images of gardening, pruning, weeding—the next best thing to a machete, which might be preferable for hacking through my psychic jungle. And how does her garden grow, I wonder?

"What's she like?" I ask Lucy. "Typhoid Mary? Is she quite contrary?"

"Ha! Not! You'll totally dig her. She's smart, and she's straightforward. She's a lot like you and me, only she's more patient, more thorough. Just as blunt, but not quite as harsh. She gets me. She'll get you, too, just call her. It'll really make a difference, you'll see."

"I'm all over it," I assure her. "I promised myself once the dust settled here I'd start psychotherapy." I'm trying to sound professional so Lucy will think I'm just going to see Dr. Shears because most psychiatrists should be on a couch at some point in their training. It's pro forma. I'm an attending now, and it's high time I join the fold. I really don't have anything wrong with me; I'm perfectly fine, perfectly sane, perfectly happy and well-adjusted. That's my story and I'm sticking to it.

If I know one thing, it's this: If I'm going to stay at Bellevue, I'll need to be in therapy to keep myself mentally healthy. I need something like a mirror to help me see how I'm doing. A self-reflecting doctor is a healthy doctor. I want Lucy to know that I understand that.

It is a Monday afternoon when Mary Shears returns my call. She is chewing something while we speak, crunching away right into the phone. I assume it's her lunch break and she has limited time to return phone calls before her next patient comes in. I forgive her this transgression, though I think it's odd that she doesn't acknowledge it and apologize.

"I got your number from Lucy," I explain. "I'm a friend of hers at Bellevue. A colleague."

"Uh-huh," she states, between swallows. I guess she wants me to go on.

"Well, I've never been in therapy before, that is, not any real therapy. I saw a therapist for a few months when I was sixteen. Anyway, I know that every psychiatrist should go through therapy at some point." I'm yammering nervously. I know she doesn't need to hear this now. She only needs to set up a time for an appointment. "So . . . I guess I'm looking for a therapist," I finally say.

"Okay," she says slowly. Maybe she is wiping her mouth? Does she have salad dressing on her chin? "I can see you next Monday, would that work for you? How's four o'clock?"

"Monday at four works great for me," I say gratefully. This will become my regular therapy slot for the next three years, the perfect time and place to reflect on my weekends at Bellevue. I need a place to unload and process all I have seen, the criminals and the crazies, and I need help understanding my cool, icy response to it all.

When I finally meet Mary at her office, a mere ten blocks from my apartment, she doesn't seem like the eating-on-the-phone type. She looks more refined, wearing a beige linen suit. She gets up to shake my hand, offers me a seat, and my eyes quickly scan the room to glean more about her. Her office is well-appointed. The predominant colors are earth tones. Like her suit, everything is a neutral shade of tan or brown: leather couch and chairs, woven throw rugs and wall-hangings, African sculptures and trinkets. I assume she is a world-traveler, bringing back proof of her adventures to adorn her end tables and walls. Her brown pocketbook is oversized, lying open on the windowsill. I see her car keys with multiple key chains and grocery tags, and guess that she drives to her office from the suburbs. She has the requisite books and journals lining the bookcases, but they do not dominate the room. Also, she has chosen not to display any diplomas or certificates.

Her hair is short and has some gray strands here and there. I'm glad she doesn't dye her hair. I have a friend in therapy who is wigged out by the frequent changes of her shrink's hairstyles and colors. How unsettling that must be, prompting the question: *How is she supposed to help me when she can't even get comfortable with her own hair?* Mary is wearing earrings that are small, and they are not dangling. Everything about her and her office is classy, tailored, understated. I like that about her immediately. Her voice is assured and low pitched.

"So, how can I help you?" she invites me to unload, and it doesn't take much more than that to open the floodgates. Just the act of being in a psychotherapist's office, sitting on the couch, has me feeling vulnerable, shaky, and weepy.

"I hate asking for help. I hate needing help. I don't need any help, actually. But I know I should undergo therapy because I'm a psychiatrist. I know it will help me to be a better doctor if I can get a handle on what my issues are, so I won't project my garbage onto the patient." This is a common understanding in psychiatry. If you are not in touch with your own trigger points, your own hot spots, you will seek them out in your patients, assigning more weight to their issues than may be appropriate. Or you will diagnose all your patients with the same label you have given

your sister or your mother or they have given you. Projection is everywhere in human behavior, a common defense, but it is never appropriate
for psychiatrists to project their pathology onto their patients.

"Where do you think this comes from, this reluctance to ask for assistance?"

"Oh, I know where it comes from already: my father," I answer simply. "His whole shtick is to be strong, capable, self-sufficient. He doesn't
ask for help, and I have always tried to win his attention by being like
him. Unconsciously, of course, at least initially." I hope that Mary will
like working with me. I am psychologically minded, forthcoming,
chatty. I want her to like me, to see that I will be interesting, yet easy. I
don't want to be any trouble.

"Although my mother is the one who always reminds me my first
sentence when I was a toddler was 'I do myself!' I've always been inde-
pendent. Actually, being the youngest of three kids, both my parents
encouraged it. It made things easier for them."

I've only been here twenty minutes, and though it may be only superficial layers of examination, we've already discussed my mother
and father, starting to blame them for my foibles. *Typical shrinkage,* I
think. And, I've already wadded up two Kleenexes. By the end of my
first session I've gone through six Kleenexes. Over the next three years,
I will judge and categorize a session by how many tissues I use. I throw
them into the woven wastebasket at the edge of the couch; they amass
like empty beer cans in a college dorm. Dead soldiers. In the first few
months, I average five a session. Then, as things die down and I get
more comfortable being the patient, I plateau at around three. Toward
the end of our work together, I will not cry at all.

When I leave Mary's office at the end of our first session, I literally
feel lighter.

"You've never had a therapist, huh? You've gone all this time keeping
so much inside you. You're carrying around an awful lot," she says near
the end.

Lady, you don't know the half of it.

Fixing a Hole

I'm a whistler, always have been. Every hospital I worked at—Temple, Mount Sinai, Bronx VA, and now here at Bellevue—I'm the doctor walking through the corridors tootling a lively tune. I whistle while I work, just like one of the seven dwarves. Doc. Or maybe Happy.

When you're the dad walking through the lobby with your empty car seat to take your new baby home, I'm the one smiling at you knowingly, congratulating you with a nod. And when you're the dad crouching down in the AES waiting room, trying to explain to your son exactly where his mother has gone, and why she won't be coming back, I'm the one who stops whistling and remembers where I am. I remind myself I can't walk around here seeming so happy; it's rude and unthinking, in front of the worried and the grieving, and they are everywhere.

It's a Sunday night in February 1997, and I'm on the inpatient unit, writing notes on the new admissions before I go down to CPEP to run the show. (This chore—how I began my shifts for the first year or two at Bellevue—was eventually reassigned to someone else.) I see familiar handwriting in one of the charts, meticulous capital letters. It's Daniel from my residency at Mount Sinai. He's at Bellevue now too, working upstairs on the wards while I'm downstairs in the CPEP. I'd heard he was working here. I haven't seen him in a year or so, but I can visualize his perfectly parted hair and Hollywood smile. His comments in the patient's medical record are punctuated by exclamation points. "The patient is now compliant with his medication!" "Patient states he is no longer suicidal!"

I finish my own charting, sans exclamatory marks, and pop my head into the nurses' lounge to say good-bye. Three women are listening to the radio; one of them tells me that some people have just been shot at the Empire State Building. We haven't heard any trauma calls on the overhead PA system (usually the shrill operator instructs the trauma surgeons, the anesthesiologists, and the chaplain to report to the ER) and there have been no disaster bells sounding. It is my first year at Bellevue and I've yet to hear them ring. I wonder how many traumas would need to come into the ER before someone considers it a disaster?

I decide to meander over to the medical ER to see if anyone needs a shrink, and get the usual jokes from the doctors and policemen about who they think needs my expertise, but the bottom line is they'll call me when they need me. The shooting victims have indeed been brought to Bellevue, but the staff is still trying to sort out who's who. There's a gaggle of uniformed police and detectives wandering around, and also a good amount of blood, if you know where to look.

I head back to the psych ER and get to work. I know I'm going to get called sooner or later to go over to the medical side to hold some hands, so I try to clean up the triage bin as best I can. Just as I'm think-ing maybe they won't need me, the social worker from the AES appears and asks me to come see the family of one of the shooting victims.

A twenty-seven-year-old rock musician, Simon, has been shot in the head. He is in critical condition, undergoing neurosurgery. He had never been to the Empire State Building before today; he was just do-ing a favor for some friends visiting the city, taking them up to see the view. His timing coincided with that of a recent Palestinian immigrant equipped with a gun and a vendetta. Simon's friend from Denmark, whose girlfriend just today told him that she is pregnant, came along with the group to the observation deck. He has been killed.

The family has been placed in a separate waiting room down the hall from the ER. Some of them are sitting on the floor outside the door, some are pacing the hallway. Most of them are crying and holding each other, their sobs wracking their bodies. Simon's two brothers with their girlfriends, an aunt and uncle, and his divorced mother and father with their respective new spouses are all waiting to hear word from the neurosurgeon. His roommates are there as well, some of whom were with him at the Empire State Building. One has witnessed the whole thing and is pretty shaken up.

The most shaken is Simon's mother.

I watch her standing in front of a wall, wailing and pounding. "Please, God, just let him live. I'll do anything."

I leave her with her supplicating grief and attempt to let the others know who I am and that I am there to help. "Lousy job you have," jokes one. I try not to take offense, but end up getting defensive about my many roles at Bellevue including grief counseling. "We're not here for grief counseling," says the aunt angrily.

Outside the room, in the hallway, Simon's mother is quivering, saying to her younger son, "I'm not strong enough for this. I know you think I am, but I'm not."

The family and friends go out of their way to describe Simon to anyone who will listen, and to each other. I notice this eulogy theme as it continues into the night. Everyone wants to talk about how wonderful he is; no one talks about themselves and their pain, their fear. The other recurring theme is the guilt. "I almost went with them. Why wasn't it me?" as opposed to the unspoken guilty relief, "Thank God it wasn't me."

A father or stepfather wants to go outside for some air, and I show him how to get to the ambulance bay, walking past big drops of blood on the floor. I wonder if he assumes the blood is Simon's. Perhaps it is the gunman's, who turned the Beretta on himself after wounding nearly a dozen others. He is pronounced dead in our trauma slot a little after eleven p.m.

There is a crowd of people gathering as I walk through the hallway to get back to CPEP. A buzz, a humming circles the crowd. It's the mayor and his disaster squad, coming to lend their support to the victims and their families. Rudy Giuliani is always good about making an appearance wherever the action is. He shakes hands, smiles, offers comforting words to the patients and their loved ones. He vows to make the city safer. One thing I'll say about Rudy, he may be a loose cannon, but he's always great in a crisis. He can pull it together better than anyone, looking calm, concerned, and strong. He's got the kind of personality that thrives when surrounded by chaos, naturally making people feel safer. The rest of America would see this side of him on 9/11.

There is a rumor being murmured by some of the hospital police that the woman the mayor is having an affair with is here; she is part of his disaster team. I've read something about a mistress recently in the *New York Post,* and I crane my neck to see if anyone wearing the blue windbreakers with the yellow block letters looks like someone he might be with.

Later in the night, I find out that Simon has survived the neurosurgery as well as the shooting. He has been very lucky in terms of the bullet's trajectory, which missed many of his brain's crucial structures. The neurosurgeon describes an entrance and exit wound above and anterior to each temple. I had assumed left to right, but the surgeon's description is "in the right and out the left." Entrance and exit wounds from bullets have a very different appearance, and I make a point of correcting my personal picture of the patient.

So now he is going to live, just like his mother begged. When she was pounding against the wall, I remember thinking, *Be careful what you wish for.* I've worked with many brain-damaged patients, people in persistent vegetative states. I worry that she'll be saddled with a son who requires total care to bathe, feed, and dress.

The thing about ER work is that it is acute. I get a tiny, traumatic slice of someone's life, and then that's it. I rarely see the patient again. Occasionally I will hear updates about a patient's condition—if it's a serious case and I've made a connection with a doctor upstairs. In Simon's case, I do hear through the grapevine that his family is visiting him regularly at the hospital, playing his band's CD for him while he is in his coma. Later, I learn that Simon has regained consciousness. Plans are made to transfer him to a rehabilitation hospital.

Twelve months later, Jeremy and I are sitting in front of our coffees at his neighborhood diner, when I see Simon's brother in a booth nearby. I recognize him immediately from our time in the waiting room. We smile and exchange pleasantries, and it isn't until he points out the bearded guy next to him who's eating his eggs that I realize it's the patient who was shot in the head, whom I never met. Simon nods at me nonchalantly and I don't really get to analyze how good his speech is, or his social graces are, for that matter. I remark to the brother how it's a miracle Simon's up and around, and he smiles and nods in reply.

Jeremy points out to me as we tuck into our own eggs, "The guy probably hears that word constantly. How it's a miracle he survived."

"But taking a bullet to the head and living to tell the tale, that really is a miracle, Jer," I try to convince him. "The only bigger miracle would be if our government could make it a little harder for a guy to buy a Beretta."

Knocking Around the Zoo

I am up on 18 North again a few weeks later, writing notes on the new patients upstairs when I notice a large bouquet of flowers on the windowsill of the nurses' station.

"What's with these?" I ask the Filipino nurse with the long, straight hair and the beautiful full lips. She is wearing denim overalls and she couldn't look any sexier if she were posing in a men's magazine. She's having an affair with one of the moonlighters, but I don't let on that I know anything about it, though he's told nearly everyone.

"They're for Daniel. He passed his boards," she explains. *His written boards,* I think to myself. His second time. I wonder if he peppered his answers with exclamation points. I know that he failed them on his first try, but I also know that this nurse doesn't know that. Because he is an attending on an inpatient ward, he hasn't told many people. I smile smugly to myself, having aced the written exam my first time out. Now I am preparing for the oral exam, which comes next, and is a killer. I guess he'll take the orals after I do.

"And you guys got him flowers. . . . That's so sweet!" I say, in perfect insincerity. I think about what a killer schmoozer he is, how easily he manipulates women with that grin of his. The nurses must fall all over him up here.

I finish my notes on the acute ward and head up to 19 West. I always save the prison ward for last. I get a testosterone rush out of standing in front of the prison gate, the bars thick with layers of glossy white paint.

"On the gate!" I bellow. I have learned this is the way the guards announce that they need the door opened for them. I lift my Bellevue ID card up to where the guard in the booth can see it, and the gate is opened electronically, noisily. I enter a small area where the officers are supposed to unload their weapons into a sand-filled metal chamber. Here I am trapped, as I must wait for the gate behind me to close completely before the one in front of me can open. Once I am through the double-gated chamber, I am in another double-gated chamber, this time longer. At one end is the log book, in front of yet another gate that leads to the forensic psych ward. At the other end of the chamber is the forensic medicine and surgery ward, for the prisoners who need medical attention. The log book is for both wards, and those who sign in reflect the many disciplines of medicine at Bellevue: orthopedic surgery, neurology, infectious disease. I pen my name legibly and print PSYCHIATRY in capital block letters. I want to represent, yo!

I am on 19 West this evening to speak to a man who has been getting a lot of press lately: a rather famous serial killer in New York City. After his recent arrest, he spent some time at Rikers Island, where it became clear to the prison psychiatrists that he was not right in the head. So they packed him up and shipped him off to us for a more thorough evaluation and one-to-one observation. He is a high profile case, and no one wants a bad outcome, thus a personal babysitter is assigned to keep an eye on him.

Although the press have not yet caught wind of this, he tried to hang himself at Rikers. Also, I see in his chart that he is reporting hearing voices; the voices told him to kill his cell-mate. Smart move, on his part, to offer up this tidbit to the Rikers shrinks. Few things will make a doctor more nervous than being responsible for a life lost.

I sit in the nurses' station of the forensic unit with my feet up on the desk. The patient's chart rests in my lap, while I munch on some stale cookies the nurses left lying around. One prisoner-patient after another comes over to the nurses' station, asking if they can have some medicine. "Can I get something to help me sleep?" "Can I get something to calm me down?" "Are you here to see me, Doc? I got this rash." I can't stay here too long, I realize, because I'm starting to attract an audience. Once the patients know a doctor is on the unit, they come out of the woodwork, hoping to have their medications changed, or their privilege status upgraded, or just hoping for someone to spend some time listening.

"I'm not here to see you guys, sorry," I explain to the gathering group. "If you need a doctor, the nurse can page the moonlighter. I'm just here to write notes on the new patients."

The alleged serial killer has already made a full confession. I heard on the news that they found his diary detailing the killings. The press is saying he is suffering from a "degenerative brain disease," whatever they think that is. If you ask me, if he's writing it all down, some part of him knows that what he's doing is terribly wrong. He is compelled to detail the killings because he needs to confess and be punished. Or else he has fetishized the experiences and wants them all meticulously documented. Either way, I'm hoping that between his confession and the diary, what I document in his chart won't change his fate much.

After reviewing his records, I muster up my courage to go search for the patient. I walk into the dayroom where there are two of "New York's Boldest," NYC Department of Corrections officers. I feel as if I'm walking into a room of caged animals; I can sense the energy level in the room amp up as I enter. Then the noises start, the catcalls, the whistling, and it reminds me of those scenes in movies when the scientist walks into her lab, into the room with the monkeys, and they all start to howl, jump, and rattle their cages.

The D.O.C. guards create a barrier between me and the other men while I interview the now-famous man at a table in the dayroom. I really just have a couple of quick questions for him and then I am out of there. I'm not easily spooked, but the forensic psych unit at Bellevue pushes even my envelope.

Wearing hospital pajamas, the prisoner is tall, thin, and bug-eyed. He is surprisingly focused, calm, and completely coherent. He is polite with me, and deferential in a way that I wasn't expecting. Well-groomed, soft-spoken, he is happy to answer my questions. I could easily spend more time with him, take him somewhere more private to do a thorough evaluation, but it isn't my job right now. I am only here to make sure he isn't currently suicidal or homicidal, and to find out if he is still hallucinating. Regardless of what I learn, I won't dare stop his one-to-one observation status. Although he is cooperative, he's not chatty in the least. Moving to a different interview spot would've been a waste of time. He offers one-word answers to most of my questions.

"Are you still hearing voices?" I ask.

"No," he answers.

"What about the suicidal thoughts? Are you still having them?"

"No."

"Are you thinking about hurting anyone else?" I ask.

"Nope," he answers simply.

"Well, is there *anything* on your mind you'd like to talk about?" I inquire sweetly, cocking my head. *Toss me a bone here, man.*

"No. I'm doing okay now," he assures me, smiling.

Great. I've got nothing.

I'm not sure what to make of him. His eye contact is good, and he isn't spewing a lot of crazy disorganized information, but he still seems a little off to me. It may just be that he isn't very bright; according to his chart, he's minimally educated, possibly even mildly retarded. I don't have a lot to go on from the interview in determining whether he is truly psychotic or not. Denying everything doesn't tell me much of anything. He could be grossly psychotic on the inside, but sealed-over and acting pretty together on the outside. Maybe that's the way serial killers usually are.

I'm just not sure how to describe his mental status in the chart, knowing it's a legal document that will be pored over by prosecutors and public defenders alike.

"Patient denies AH, SI, HI," I write succinctly, using the standard abbreviations for auditory hallucinations, suicidal ideation, and homicidal ideation. Then I write what I always do when I haven't gotten anything juicy in a three-minute conversation: "No gross evidence of psychosis currently, though brevity of interview precludes full assessment. Continue current level of care."

Bor-ing.

Why are the notorious bad guys in the news always so dull when I finally get a crack at them? As the years roll by at Bellevue, this will become a recurring pattern. The more hyped-up they are in the press, the saner they seem when I finally get to sit down with them for an interview. Well, maybe not sane, exactly. They're deeply troubled, but mostly, when I scratch the surface, there isn't much underneath. They're almost always undereducated or borderline retarded, and they're often quite childlike. Talking to a psychotic killer, I will learn after a few years at the hospital, is a lot like talking to a dumb kid, only it's more pathetic. With a kid at least you have a sense of optimism about his future.

This prisoner, though he is not one to brag, has left a wake of carnage that the city won't easily forgive or forget. I appreciate that I have a chance to speak to him, however briefly. Bellevue will always be kind in affording me these opportunities. It is one of the reasons I came here, and one of the reasons I stay.

I leave the prison gates and head for the relative freedom of CPEP to start my shift.

Little Earthquakes

Two nurses and a few psych techs are standing around a stretcher in the shower room. A woman has come in by ambulance from a crack house and is in desperate need of bathing. Her hair is sticky and covered with dirt; she is speckled with mud and feces, and from what we can tell, semen. She has scratches all along her back and buttocks, and bruises on the insides of her thighs.

She is either still high on cocaine or a combination of drugs, or she is out of her mind from trauma—I can't tell which. While she is being scrubbed clean, she arches her back, and opens her mouth wide toward the head of the stretcher, jutting her chin toward the ceiling. She keeps making these openmouthed sucking motions, and groaning rhythmically. Groaning and gulping, absentmindedly, automatically, as if she's been doing that for hours already.

"Julie," says Nancy, in her froggy voice, "I think she been raped." Nancy is my very favorite nurse. Love Nancy. With her ample bosom and her gap-toothed grin, she is my warm, welcoming, and accepting auntie, and I would do just about anything for her.

"Maybe we shouldn't be washing the evidence off her?" I wonder aloud. "Should we send her to AES for a rape kit?" It is standard procedure: If someone reports a rape they are sent to the medical ER to be examined. A rape kit is a forensic physical, a way of examining a sexual assault victim with a fine-tooth comb, literally. It can be traumatic for the patient, resonating with the assault itself, but it's the best way to collect DNA evidence to assist in prosecution. The vagina and anus are swabbed for semen samples, and the pubic hair is combed for the rapist's pubic hairs. Also, pictures are taken of the bruises, abrasions, and any other physical signs of the attack.

"I don't think she was in any shape to identify anyone," Nancy surmises. "Plus, I imagine she did it for the drugs. You know how these things go. It's best we clean her up, let her sleep. She looks like she been through enough. I say let it be."

I suppose she's right. I watch my coworkers, my friends, tend to this woman, lovingly washing away the dirt, the grime, and the evidence of the crime. I am touched by the scene, the symbolism of the water, the baptism. I hope it washes her clean, inside and out. I hope she can't remember a blessed thing, unlike our other rape patient in the CPEP.

That woman, who is in the EOU, was attacked just a few blocks from here under the FDR, the highway next to the hospital. She was hit on the back of the head and tackled by two guys. They took her wallet and sexually assaulted her, but then the cops drove up. The two guys ran in two different directions. One of them ran across the highway and was hit by a car. The ambulance brought him to Bellevue, where he was rushed into the trauma slot. The other guy was caught by the cops and taken to central booking.

My friend Jude, one of the AES attendings, calls me with an update. I'm always happy to talk to him. He's fun to flirt with, and usually flirts back even more insistently than I do, even though he knows about Jeremy.

"Hey, Jude," I coo.

"Hey, bulldog. You know that rape victim you have over there?" he asks.

"You wanna narrow it down for me, lovey? I got more than one in the area."

"Yeah, lessee . . . white woman, mid-thirties? What's her name, Jackson? Johnson? Something like that . . ."

"Johansen," I say, exaggerating a Swedish accent. "Jah, she's still here. What about her?"

"Maybe you want to let her know her attacker didn't make it. He died in the slot."

"Ouch. Well, sorry you lost one, pal, but maybe not so sorry it was this one in particular, huh? Okay, I'll let her know. I guess you really are supposed to look both ways before you cross the street. Even if you're running from the cops."

"Turns out . . . so, uh . . . maybe I'll come by later to tuck you in, huh?" he teases.

This is a long-standing joke between us: our mutual attraction, and also the fact that I sleep through a good chunk of my overnight shift, while he works every minute of his. Later that night, when my pager goes off with a callback number of 6969696969, I will assume it is him and roll over, settling back to sleep with a smile.

"Tuck me in . . . I wish," I sigh dramatically. "Are you wearing those light blue scrubs that drive me wild?"

"I am, indeed!"

And on it goes. I hang up the phone and go to the EOU where Ms. Johansen is lying in bed, curled up in the fetal position with her back to the door.

I enter her room quietly, not sure if she's sleeping or not, and lean over her to get a look at her eyes. She is staring at the wall, barely blinking, breathing shallowly. "Hi," I say softly, tentatively. "How are you feeling?"

She rolls over to see who is addressing her. "Mostly numb," she answers. "My head hurts, still, but the anti-anxiety medicine is working pretty well. I finally stopped shaking. I can't stop seeing their faces, though. It doesn't seem to matter if I close my eyes or if they're open. I keep replaying what happened."

"That's perfectly normal after a trauma," I explain. "It's called intrusive recollections. It goes away in a few days, usually." Can I give her any useful advice? "Don't try to fight the memories. You really can't. Just let them play out and know it's your brain's way of dealing with what happened. It won't go on forever."

She sits up, moves her pillow to behind her back, and motions for me to sit on the edge of the bed.

"I have some news for you, sort of," I begin. "One of the attackers, the one who got hit by the car on FDR?"

"Yeah?"

"He was brought here to Bellevue, to what is called the trauma slot, where critically injured patients are worked on by the ER doctors." I pause to give her a minute to process what I have just said, and to brace for what's coming next. "He died."

"Okay," she says easily. "But the other one's still alive?"

"Right. As far as I know, he got taken by the police to central booking, you know, to get fingerprinted, mug shot taken, all that. They'll keep him there until he gets arraigned. They call it the tombs, where the prisoners wait to see the judge. I guess it's kind of a creepy place."

"I hope it is creepy," she says. "I hope he's scared, and can't breathe and has the same tight chest I have. He should spend the rest of his life behind bars."

I know this won't happen. Even if he gets convicted, which is always a huge if, they don't give rapists life in prison as a rule. The pot dealers get longer sentences half the time. Don't get me started.

"So, you try and rest now, okay? Do you want me to send in a nurse with some more medicine so you can sleep?"

"Could you? I'd really appreciate that. I just want to turn my brain off. Do you have anything that would do that?"

"I've got just the thing," I say convincingly, though I'm not sure exactly what I'm going to order when I get to the nurses' station. I rise off her bed and the door opens.

"Dr. Holland, can you come to my office for a minute?" It's Rita, who rarely leaves the clerk's office, and even more rarely enters the patients' rooms. "Sorry to interrupt, Ms. Johansen," she says pleasantly.

I follow Rita to the clerk's office, curious as all hell. "What's going on? Why didn't you just overhead page me?" I look around her desk. Hundreds of pennies, nickels, dimes, and quarters have been segregated and organized. Wads of wrinkled bills are stacked according to denomination. She is vouchering property for a recently admitted patient, a panhandler. Her gloves are black from counting the money.

"I did page you. I guess you didn't hear me. Too busy having your little heart-to-heart in there."

"Well, did you hear? One of the rapists died in the slot."

"I know. Everybody knows. The AES clerk called me and I told Nancy. But you are not going to believe this."

"What?"

"The cops just brought in a pre-arraignment. I was going through his wallet to look for a health insurance card. You'll never guess what I found. Are you ready?"

She is milking it a little, adding to the suspense. She is holding a driver's license in her hand, but it's turned around so I can't see the picture and name. She flips it over and hands it to me.

"Leah Johansen," I read. Why does this guy have my patient's driver's license? Was her wallet stolen? "Wait a minute. You can't be serious. This is the other rapist?" my voice is loud. Rita shushes me. "You're kidding me! They brought this guy here? What for? Why?"

"He's on Prozac and needs to be cleared," explains Rita.

"This is too much! Jesus, what are the chances?"

"Well, he's arrested in our borough and he's on psych meds. So here he is," she says. "Nancy's trying to keep him in the nondetainable area so Johansen can't see him."

"Oh, shit! I didn't even think of that! She can't see him. She'll go nuts. And he can't see her either! I mean, who knows what he'll do if he sees her? Do you think he knows she's here? I mean, does he know where she is? You think he has any idea?"

"How the hell should I know? Get a load of you! Why are you getting so worked up?"

"I don't know, Rita. It's just . . . this is crazy, don't you think? I mean, it's another one of those 'you can't make this shit up,' you know?"

"I know. She gets mauled by two guys. She's brought to Bellevue, a basket case. Thug number one runs into traffic and is brought to the nearest hospital, us. Criminal number two gets caught by the cops, and needs to be cleared by a shrink. Bring him to Bellevue! Why not? Everyone else is here?!" She's laughing, but her eyes are wet. It's sweet. She knows: It's funny, but it's not so funny.

I go see the criminal and give him about two minutes of my time. He is shifting his weight from leg to leg, probably in withdrawal from opiates, but his greasy hair and pimpled complexion suggest meth. "Are you hearing voices? Are you suicidal? Do you feel like hurting anyone?"

No, no, and no.

I take the cop aside and explain the situation. I give him the two forms he needs from me, and he is happily out the door. I can fill in the rest of the paperwork later.

Don't Let It Bring You Down

I got the letter two days ago informing me that I have failed my oral exams to become board-certified in psychiatry. I passed the written exam a year earlier, soon after I got to Bellevue, but the oral portion with a live patient, usually taken a year after residency, is notoriously difficult to pass, with nearly a fifty-percent fail rate. This information does nothing to make me feel better. I am devastated and I can't stop crying for one solid day. *Other people fail exams, not me,* I think to myself. *How could this possibly happen?* Here's how:

I walk into this small office in an outpatient clinic, and there are two male examiners in the corner behind a desk. The patient to be examined is in a chair in front of the desk, and there's an empty chair for me. I sit down and introduce myself and right off, I'm transfixed by her appearance. It really throws me off. She's got very close-cropped jet-black hair, dark eye makeup on the lid above and also circled underneath, and she's very pale. Maybe it's her makeup, or maybe she only eats white food, who the hell knows, but she is ashen. With multiple piercings and tattoos and this vicious glare, her whole look is totally goth and dramatic. I should've been tipped off right there, but I was laser-focused on doing my job—and not getting thrown—so I didn't stop and tune in to her, and think, *How should I play this?*

I keep to my game plan and start with all my usual background questions, trying to keep it superficial: Do you have any medical problems? Are you allergic to anything? What meds are you taking? I'm not getting into her symptoms at all. This isn't the way most people start the interview. It certainly isn't the recommended way, which is that you let the patient free-float and tell you all their problems for the first five minutes.

No, siree, I had a format I wanted to follow, my way of efficiently building a database, and I wanted her to go along with it.

She interrupts my rapid-fire style. "I'm done answering your questions." She looks me right in the eye, and says, "I don't know where I am right now. I don't really know *what* I am. I mean, I don't even know if I'm a human being!"

I respond calmly, matching her intimidating gaze, staring her down. "You are in the outpatient clinic, you *are* a human being, and I have a lot more questions to ask you, so let's just continue."

It's the worst thing in the world to say, I know now. She handed me a bunch of symptoms on a silver platter and I tossed the tray, toppling them all. I was just trying to keep her on track, on my schedule. I had only thirty minutes to get her whole story. This was *my* exam. I didn't feel like this was about her. I figured she volunteered for this because she wanted to be part of the process, she wanted to help me pass.

I'm an idiot.

It just goes downhill from there. I should've realized the only way to win the examiners over was to win her over, but I guess I thought I could be a star in their eyes and still afford to be an asshole in hers.

A big part of what you are judged on in the boards is the ability to establish rapport with the patient. You need those points to pass. But somehow, when faced with a bad situation, I just imploded. I tried to out-macho the patient. Bad idea.

I see that I'm going to have to work on all of this with Mary before I take the exam again. We've got to soften me up somehow, and fast. This steamroller cowboy thing isn't getting me anywhere. Except . . .

After hearing about my failure, Jeremy makes me a card to cheer me up. He has Photoshopped an old picture of me from my rock-and-roll days, onstage with my band in tight jeans and a white tank top, my nipples clearly visible. I am wearing dark sunglasses, microphone in hand, and my mouth is wide open.

Below the picture, he has written a caption:

Julie, you pass your orals with me every time.

Piggies

When the weather turns frigid, the homeless head indoors, crowding the CPEP beds and perfuming the area with the piercing stench of fungus. People assume the odor would be worse in the summer, but it is always considerably more unbearable in the winter. Patients who live on the street wear multiple layers, sweatshirts and coats that trap the aromas of the body. As they peel each layer off, the smell intensifies, sometimes becoming overpowering enough to make my eyes water, or even to make me gag. When all I want to do is run in the other direction, it gets a lot harder to be therapeutic and caring toward the patients.

Still, when I greet a new patient in the nondetainable area who has matted-down hair, and bugs in his clothing, smelling of urine, sweat, and feces, even if I can't help but turn my head away, stifling a "PHEW!" I am careful not to say anything. It's not his fault. There is nowhere to shower in the city but the shelters, and most of the street people avoid the shelter system like a bear avoids a trap. There are too many rules, addicts, alcoholics, scammers, and lunatics. Things get stolen constantly and people get assaulted at random hours, so no one can ever truly relax or sleep.

This weekend at CPEP has been hell, and it has taught me a valuable lesson: Take time off in January. That's when the census starts to creep up through the twenties, day after day. Tonight, not only are there nearly thirty people in the area, but they are impressively sick. Many of the patients need wrist and ankle restraints. The process of restraining a patient requires anywhere from four to eight staff members: usually CPEP psych techs and nurses, who are big women, and hospital police, who are smaller men. (Sometimes the sizes and genders are reversed; it depends who's on shift.) Each staffer takes a limb, and one person stands near the head to oversee the procedure. A doctor is supposed to be present at all restrainings, trying to get the patient to calm down, explaining, "This is only a temporary procedure, until you have better control over yourself. We're just trying to keep everyone safe." It's usually a bit of a mess, with a lot of swearing, grunting, and threatening.

On Sunday, the flurry of aggression that necessitates one man to be restrained sets off another patient who is escalating. Angry that he is being admitted involuntarily, he is screaming at me and kicking the wall. I try to get him to calm down, encouraging him, "Please, try to keep it together so you don't get tied up," but he is unable to contain himself. Like a ripple effect in a Rockette line of dancers, five people end up getting restrained over the course of one Sunday afternoon. I wish I were home watching football, instead of at work watching wrestling.

As I fill out the paperwork on the five patients, I am multitasking. Writing and listening, I nod my head to confirm the information is reaching my brain as Nancy tells me about a case that has just come in: a former corrections officer who used to work for D.O.C., who is now a homeless man. He has been arrested for jumping a subway turnstile, which is how we get a good chunk of our homeless patients these days. While in his cell, he defecated on himself and threw his feces at the guards, so NYPD brought him to us.

It becomes clear, once he has been interviewed, that this man is completely out of his mind. He has some sort of psychosis; whether brought on by drugs or mental illness, I can't yet say, but what *is* said is an oft-spoken line by Nancy. "He ain't goin' nowhere but up." Unquestionably, he needs to be admitted to the prison psychiatric ward upstairs. In order for him to go up he needs to undergo a physical exam, a chest X-ray, and an EKG. He also needs his blood drawn for routine testing. All of these tests require the patient to be cooperative and lie still, or else to be sedated.

Although the former corrections officer acquiesces to the EKG and the chest X-ray, the psych tech informs me that he is refusing to allow his blood to be taken. I leave the relative comfort and safety of the nurses' station to find the patient.

I give him my usual shtick. "Here's the deal, sir," I begin. "You're going to have your blood taken. It's a requirement for the admission. It is up to you whether this happens with you tied up and sedated or freely moving and cooperating." In psychiatry, this is the oldest trick in the book, the old "choice-no-choice" paradigm. This gives the patient the illusion of control over a situation, offering him a choice that implies freedom, when really there is none. I had used the technique earlier with another man who required a bed upstairs by saying, "You're going to be admitted to the hospital. Would you like to be a voluntary or an involuntary patient?" You'd be surprised how often this works, especially with toddlers.

The former C.O., no dummy, is not falling for it. He tells me, "There is no fucking way you are taking my blood. Period."

I have seen patients who are hesitant about blood draws. Sometimes it's a needle phobia, but other times it's something more delusional. "Are you afraid of needles?" I ask.

"No."

"Do you think there's something special in your blood that you'll lose if we take a few teaspoons?" I've had psychotic patients who are deathly afraid of losing some sort of vital power if their blood is removed.

He stares at me blankly, either unable to fathom what I'm trying to get at, or perhaps acutely afraid that I can read his mind. I can't tell, but if it's the latter, he's masking the suspicion well. He doesn't look very paranoid, but he is dead set against the blood draw.

The arresting officer is hanging out in the detainable area watching football. He is near the patient and overhears our short exchange. "Can I have some time alone with my prisoner?" he asks me. He rolls the former D.O.C. officer's wheelchair down the hall and then begins to threaten this patient with various forms of aggression, beating the hell out of him, slamming his face into something, and other things I can't hear fully. I am alarmed at how quickly the cop goes from zero to sixty. There is no small talk, no chitchat, no cajoling, just immediate threats of violence. The cop isn't getting anywhere with this tactic; he is, however, getting progressively redder in the face.

I know how these things go, and I know that we will eventually have to tie our patient down and sedate him in order to obtain his blood. The lab technician is waiting patiently along with a number of CPEP staff and hospital police who are lined up along one wall, assuming we'll have to do a restraint, while the man from NYPD issues his threats at the man formerly from D.O.C. down the hall.

I finally intervene, mostly because I know the lab tech waiting to draw his blood is getting antsy. She has other patients to get to in other parts of the hospital.

As I get closer to the two of them, I can hear the NYPD cop yelling, "I'm gonna pull down your pants and pull on your balls until you howl if you don't start cooperating with the doctor."

I step in and tell the officer as calmly as I can, "That's all right. We're just going to restrain him. It'll be easier for everyone."

After the patient is cuffed to the stretcher, the arresting officer makes a big show out of snapping on a pair of gloves, making motions to pull down the man's pants, licking his lips, saying, "I hope your balls are big and juicy. This is going to hurt and I'm going to enjoy it."

Picking my jaw off the floor, I ask the officer in an overly polite manner, "Um, actually, sir, could you please just step away from the patient? We're going to take over now."

Throughout the melee that ensues, which requires eight people to restrain him, a sheet to be placed over his mouth so he cannot spit or bite, and his arms and legs to be tied to the stretcher, the patient yells and curses, threatening to come back one day and kill us all. "I'll do each one of you. I'll fuck you all up. I'll fucking kill you, and I'll fuck up your cars, too, and then you'll know it's me that did it." Soon after his blood is taken, the man falls asleep from the sedating medication.

The arresting officer takes off his gloves and retreats from the patient, acting as if he has helped us with the restraint process. He takes me aside and explains to me in a stage whisper, "I hope that I didn't offend you with my language. These are techniques we use to get criminals to comply." His language is stilted, formal and rehearsed. He sounds like he's reading from an official guide to police behavior. He reaches out to shake my hand, implying to me that we are on the same team, the restraining team.

I am repulsed. I try not to roll my eyes or grimace as I say to him in a complicit tone, "I totally understand. Whatever works," and shake his sweaty hand. *Nice technique, dude. The ol' pull-your-juicy-balls threat. Worked like a charm. And that last scene about your enjoyment, in front of a standing-room audience? Bravo.*

I cannot look him in the eye. I walk away thinking how he is a power-hungry, maniacal little weakling, and how much I resent his aligning himself with me.

Not for the first time, I find myself reflecting on the sadomasochism involved in being a cop or a corrections officer. How incredibly homo-erotic it all is: the nightsticks with the handles shaped like dildos, the handcuffs, the shiny black leather boots, the men putting other men into cages, the bondage, the discipline, the dungeons. The anal rape be-tween prisoners, or between the cops and the criminals. Which came first: the fetish or the job?

And how did a corrections officer snap so hard? How did he slide from D.O.C. to homeless psychotic? Was he already flirting with the edge of reality when he took the job? Was he seriously psychiatrically ill and they missed it, or was he snorting mountains of cocaine when he was off duty? And will this city cop, the supposedly sane one, ever become as insane and violent as my patient? He can't act that sadistic all the time, right? Does he have control over how he turns on and off that homoerotic rage?

When I can't get the patients to do what I want, it drives me crazy. I get angry. Sometimes I even get mean. I've seen how I act and it's high time I spoke to Mary about it. Seeing the cop get so nasty, I was embar-rassed for him. I don't ever want to be like that, controlling yet impo-tent if I don't get my way with a patient.

Or am I already like that? Is this why I can't stop thinking about him?

I'm counting on Mary to help shed some light on this.

I Should've Known Better

Mary and I spend several sessions trying to tease apart the sadistic impulses I'm experiencing at CPEP. Some of the analysis is easy: I turn my fear into aggression, my default position is to act like a hard-ass to hide my dismay at the casualties being wheeled to my ER. And then my best defense turns into a good offense.

"I was rewarded by my father for being a tough guy in my childhood," I explain. "I remember him standing in his underwear. The garage door was open, and he was yelling at me. I remember thinking, *He's in his underwear for the whole neighborhood to see, but he doesn't care about that, because he's too busy yelling at me.* I was in kindergarten, and I had run home from the bus stop before the bus came, because some of the bigger kids there were making fun of me. I came to him crying, begging for his help, and he was very clear with me: I had to go back there and fight my own battles. He was not going to fight them for me. But he was turning me away in a disgusted manner."

Mary and I decide that most of the macho behavior, my biggest defense at my job, comes back to my proving myself to my father. Growing up, I did fight my own battles, and I became a bit of a bully in the process. I wound up the winner, more often than not. But there were others who did not fare as well as I, especially my two sisters.

"You know, the way you paint it, it sounds to me like you have survivor guilt, to some extent, because you figured out how to get your father's love and attention, which was in short supply in your house, and you ended up in a better position than your sisters."

"Not only was my strength and power rewarded, my father admired self-sufficiency. I could win his admiration by being stoic and cheerful, pretending that I didn't need him or anyone else to do anything for me. It became a huge part of my persona. I'm Julie, the girl who doesn't need anything from anyone. I can do it all myself. Why do you think it was so hard for me to start therapy?

"Some of my earliest memories are of him rejecting me when I was acting needy. Like this one time, I remember being in a car with my parents. I'm sitting between them in the front seat, being incredibly thirsty, and making noises with my mouth to imply just how thirsty I am, when my dad screams at me to be quiet. My mom defends me, telling him I'm just thirsty, but he's upset that I am making so much noise about it. He'd prefer I suffer in silence, which is definitely how he does it."

"So, how did that make you feel?" asks Mary.

I hate that stupid question. It's the hardest part of psychotherapy for me. I can never quite put myself back there entirely, to feel what the little girl was feeling. "Well, I guess I remember feeling really sad and rejected, that he wasn't sympathetic, not just that, but that he was disdainful of me in that state of need. I felt his disdain, his revulsion."

"And now? Where do you stand?"

"It's second nature for me now, to deny that I need anything."

"Hmm . . . I'm just wondering how this might play out at the hospital. You're surrounded by people in a state of need, but you don't reject them, do you?" Mary asks.

"Well, that's complicated. I think there are times when I do, when I treat them just the way my dad treated me. But I took this job, I went into psychiatry, really, because I wanted to help people in need. I wanted to fix it so they felt better. I respond immediately to people who need something—anything—impulsively. I want to plug the hole. Like, I have to stifle this impulse to help people carry their grocery bags in my apartment building, or if I'm in line at the store and someone is short some money, I'll always think about volunteering to pay. Even on the street, I'll hear someone complain about how they can't get somewhere, I'll think, *I have a car you can borrow.* I don't say it, thank God, but I find myself thinking it. If I see someone shivering on the street, I have an impulse to give them the coat off my back. It's pathological, right? I have a neurotic impulse to help people?"

"I'm not sure I'd say it's pathological. It's interesting, and as long as you're thinking it, and not constantly acting on being the Good Samaritan, I'm not sure there's anything wrong with having that impulse. It's probably one of the things that makes you a good doctor. You have a genuine desire to make things better for other people."

"Well, that's true enough. It is one of the reasons I went to work at Bellevue. I wanted to help the homeless schizophrenics I saw on the street when I was a kid. It's almost like I'm trying to make sure no one else ends up needy like I was. I'm trying to avoid the whole situation. It's all just projection, isn't it? Me gratifying their needs because I want my own fulfilled?"

"Right. The flip side of it is, you're trying to make sure no one else ends up in a state of need, which you find intolerable."

Mary, as usual, seems to get exactly what I'm saying. It feels good to be understood, and my mood starts to ease as I keep talking.

"Luckily, at Bellevue, it works out fine because I have the tools to help, I can plug the holes and give people what they want, to some extent. The problem comes when they're intensely, dramatically needy, and I can't fix everything for them. I think I go into 'reject mode' then. I want them away from me. I turn into my dad, I guess, disdaining them for making too much noise about being thirsty. But also, I'm uncomfortable. I don't want to be confronted with my ineptness, with my impotence in the face of their illness."

"Do you think this is some form of projected self-hatred?" asks Mary, cutting to the chase. I like that. Other therapists would wait around for the patient to arrive at her own conclusions, but Mary offers it up herself for our discussion.

"I think it is, yes. It's pretty much as simple as that, right? Dad hates me needy. I hate myself needy. I hate you needy."

Good psychotherapy is like an archaeological dig. We spend our sessions "digging in the dirt," to quote Peter Gabriel, to find the places in my past where I was wounded and have scarred over. They are tender areas, well-guarded, inhabiting terrain that is difficult to navigate. I feel as though Mary and I are colleagues on an excavation, trying to make sense of a large, puzzling site. We poke around until we find an item, dust it off, study it, and together we learn how it fits into the scheme of what we have already uncovered.

It has been enlightening, to say the least. I am enjoying our work together and hope that she is too. Mary is trying to help me to be a better person, and I'm desperately hoping that will translate into my becoming a better doctor . . . or at least less of a tyrant at CPEP.

Papa Don't Preach

Sunday night and I have the opportunity to speak with an eighteen-year-old girl who has just killed her baby. That's how the cop presents it to me, but later it's clarified: She's just been arrested for the death of her baby, which occurred two weeks ago. Being the attending in charge, I can assign the case to a resident, or even a medical student, but I choose to take the case myself. I've never talked to anyone who's done this, and I'm curious. I'll admit it: Part of the appeal of psychiatry for me is the voyeurism—I am allowed to ask anything. The standard rules of social etiquette do not apply.

For a pre-arraignment evaluation, I only need assess suicidality or dangerousness secondary to psychosis, whether the prisoner is safe to be in police custody and can behave appropriately in front of the judge. The shrinks at Bellevue set the bar pretty high, though. Whenever we can, we try to turn them around, these prisoners-turned-patients, and send them back with NYPD to be arraigned. This will likely be one of those times.

Initially, the girl told the police that she'd woken up in the morning and the baby had been facedown in the crib, presumed to be asleep, but actually dead. When they returned to her home for questioning after the autopsy revealed suffocation, she admitted that she smothered her baby with a pillow.

"What happened?" I ask.

"He wouldn't stop crying. I fed him and changed him, but he

wouldn't stop. I finally put a pillow over his face to stop it. When I pulled the pillow away, he was still breathing . . . but kind of like little breaths. And he wasn't crying anymore, so I put him in his crib and I went to bed. I needed to sleep. When I got up in the morning, he was dead."

"So you didn't mean to kill him."

"No." She begs me with her eyes to believe her.

She has no psychiatric history to speak of. She is not currently psychotic, nor has she ever been. She may be eighteen, but she acts and talks like she is much younger—a guileless child. The main issue is this: Can she handle where she's at and what's coming next or will she fall apart and kill herself?

She is clearly distressed and feeling guilty, yet won't go so far as to say that she is suicidal, or even depressed.

"What happens now? What should I do next?" she asks me, reading my mind.

"I'm not sure how to answer that. If you leave here, you'll go with the police to get arraigned in front of the judge. Then they'll either release you on bail, or they'll keep you in custody, I guess."

"In jail? In a cell?" she asks nervously.

"I guess so, yes," I answer. "Unless it seems like you're too sick to go with the police, then I would send you to a hospital psych ward for a while."

"But I'm not crazy. I just don't know what to do now, is all . . ." her voice trails off before switching gears. "Am I going to be in the newspapers, do you think?" she asks, her voice a different tone.

"I have no idea. Why?" I ask.

"Because I'm afraid my baby daddy's family is going to come down on me and my parents."

"You're worried about what they'll do?"

"I should have to pay for what I done," she explains to me. "Maybe I should be dead too?" She asks me this question as if I would answer it. I wonder if her alluding to her death being an equal retribution for the baby's death qualifies as suicidality. Can I safely send her out to be arraigned if she's thinking in these terms? After asking her some more questions, I am assured that she has no real intention of trying to kill herself. She's just at a loss for what she is meant to do now. She's like a small child who knows that she's in trouble, nervously awaiting her punishment. Over time, I bet she'll probably put herself through worse than anything the DA can dish up.

"I wish I could just rewind my life by a year."

I imagine she's thinking that maybe she should never have had the baby, but I don't ask that, and she does not offer it up. "What about the father? The baby's daddy?" I ask. "Where was he when this happened?"

"He left me to go back to his girlfriend." She finally starts to cry. She wipes her eyes with the back of her hand. "He already has a baby with her."

Now I need to shift gears, hoping if I change the subject, she'll stop thinking about how her boyfriend left her and the baby to fend for themselves. Her tears began here, so I know this is a hot spot. I'm already convinced that if he had stayed around, the baby would still be alive, but it's not my place to get into that with her. I don't want her to fall apart on me now. I'm hoping I can send her out to be arraigned, and I'm worried if we keep talking about her boyfriend, she's going to crumble.

"I need to talk to someone who knows you, like a parent or a family member who can tell me a little bit about your medical history." She gives me her father's phone number and I call him to verify that she has no history of prior suicide attempts.

"I am not saying anything to anyone until I speak to a lawyer," he barks.

He's probably already been on the phone with the police, or the DA's office, or both. Maybe he's being hounded by reporters already; I'm not sure how quickly the press catches wind of a story like this.

"Sir, I understand your situation, but I am her doctor right now. I'm not a prosecutor. My purpose here is to make sure she's not in any danger. Can you at least verify that she has no history of self-harm?"

"I'm not telling you anything until I talk to a lawyer . . . but . . . if you are her doctor, could you maybe give her something to calm her down?" He has no idea how calm she is, relatively speaking.

Then I hand her the phone so she can talk to her dad. I'm not supposed to let prisoners use the phone, but I don't stop to think too much about this. There's some part of me who wants to see the little scared girl talking to her daddy, to see if she'll be comforted or criticized. She is holding the phone but can no longer get out any words. She listens to her dad and nods her head, her body heaving as she clutches the phone, her voice quivering as she tries to slow down her breathing enough to tell him that she's okay.

I take the phone from her hands, and I find her a box of tissues. I ask the nurses to give her some Ativan, an oral sedative, and I quickly complete the paperwork that will allow her to leave with the detectives. She needs to be fingerprinted, photographed, and arraigned. My time with her is over.

I walk out to the nondetainable area to make sure she has gotten her medication and that the police have their paperwork for the judge. The detectives look sharp; they're wearing suits and ties. I am used to seeing blue-uniformed officers in the ER, but these guys came from the station where the questioning had been, and not from the street.

"You boys look pretty dapper this evening," I comment.

"Sure," one of them says, "we're going to be in the paper tomorrow."

The next morning, as I sift through the newspapers at Starbucks, I see a picture of the three of them, the two detectives and my patient, in the *New York Post*.

They are all smiling.

Come Together

I think of my job as a psychiatrist as being, in many ways, a seduction. Getting the patient to align with me is a major part of what I do in the ER. I use my feminine wiles to have my way with the patients, convincing them that what I have to offer is valid, or at least attractive, and that they can trust me. Sometimes, I can talk a patient down, lulling him enough to avoid getting restrained. Other times, I will sit across from him almost as if on a date, inviting him to open up and tell me about himself. My endgame is for him to divulge what is really going on, where it hurts, and to admit that he needs help.

My powers of persuasion come in handy out front, too, in the non-detainable area, when the patients are first brought to the CPEP by the NYPD or EMS. I aim to be as enticing to the cops as a doughnut. I feel like I keep Bellevue in business by encouraging these guys to come around again and again. Flirting at my job is my pleasure and my prerogative. Everyone seems happy to join in. Being around ambulance workers and policemen, there's this heady mix of testosterone and adrenaline, and I feel fine.

This kind of male-dominated scenario reminds me of med school, my third-year surgery rotation: It was summer in Philadelphia and humid. We were turgid, sweating animals, jockeying for sexual position among ourselves, rubbing up against each other in the OR, the ER, and the call-rooms. The ratio worked in my favor: There was basically a gaggle of good-looking guys in loose-fitting scrubs, and there was me.

All of the surgeons were men a little older than I was, some married, some single, but, as far as I could tell, they were all horny. The flirting and sexual innuendos were nonstop.

We were in the OR; I got to scrub in on an emergency appendectomy. I held the plastic vacuum tube in the body cavity to collect the draining blood. The third-year resident told me, "Suck." I moved the suction tube to where he pointed, where fresh blood was pooling. "That's good, now suck here. She's quite talented at this, isn't she, doctor?" he joked to the second-year resident. I was humiliated, blushing, but still, I was excited that they found me attractive enough to make sexual jokes. Later, the surgical residents paged me out of a sound sleep to come to the ER, and when I got there, they were telling me how to put a catheter in a man's penis, laughing while they instructed me to "Hold it like it's your own. Yeah, grab it like you mean it!"

They killed me, these guys. Maybe not individually, but as a group, they had it all: smarts, humor, balls, looks. It was mostly a question of which one to pick. I'd made a bet with a girlfriend of mine, another third-year who'd also started off with surgery, to see who could have sex with a resident in a call-room first. It was a competition I intended to win.

I was in a service elevator, alone with my senior resident, as he explained how to place a central line in a patient. This is a procedure involving sliding a needle under the clavicle, the horizontal bone at the top of the chest. He told me how to puncture the subclavian artery, as he slowly, gently touched my shoulder, sliding his fingers along the length of my clavicle, his palm edging closer to my breast, his face pressed to mine, smiling slyly, not shyly, while his hands were busy working overtime. It was three in the morning and we were wearing scrubs, which pretty much felt like we were staying up all night wearing pajamas. The Temple scrubs were a faded shade of maroon, of blood, worn down by years of industrial-strength laundering, and they felt smooth and soft against our skin. There were only two paper-thin layers of material between our two bodies, making it oh-so-painfully obvious that he was as aroused as I. The urge to grind my pulsing pelvis right up against his was nearly overpowering, but he continued to explain central line placement. Did he think I was paying attention to what he was saying? Did he think there was any blood left in my brain?

The surgeons and I spent July and August together, sleeping in the call-rooms or working all night and greeting the dawn. That's one of the things I'll never forget about that summer. Few surgeons on call ever see the sun going down, but oh, those sunrises! In the early mornings of my overnights, whether I was in the ER, or the surgeon's lounge finishing up from the OR, or the intensive care units of the hospital, more than once I managed to catch a glimpse out of some east-facing window of a spectacular, honeyed mango and papaya sunrise. No matter what mayhem went on the night before, no matter how many people were shot or stabbed or died in a car crash, and no matter what psychological trauma their families were buried under, the sun would rise gloriously the next day. I remember gazing out those windows, marveling at the impassivity of the universe: The cycle continued, bar nothing.

The summer went by in a flash, and my own cycle continued: sex, death, sunrise, sex, death, sunrise. I was totally sleep-deprived, buzzing electric. With the surging adrenaline of the ER traumas, the resulting emergency surgeries, and me encircled by men all summer long, by the end of it I was in a permanent state of arousal. The whole idea of surgery was now so charged with sexual tension, I reflexively lubricated at the sight of surgical scrubs.

Over the next two years of my clinical rotations, I slept with an orthopedic surgeon who had pierced his own nipples, I bedded two attendings during one ER rotation, and I had a steamy affair with a married neurosurgeon. Scrubs, scrubs, scrubs, scrubs. Just like a trained animal, if I saw a pair, I could not help but become aroused.

The whole Pavlovian conditioning persists throughout my time at Bellevue as well. Guys I would never look at twice cause me to salivate if they're in scrubs. The white coat does nothing for me, but put a man in a pair of reversible cotton pants that tie around the waist, and I am all his.

I am hanging out in the CPEP; it's not very busy, and Paul, one of the doctors from the medical ER, has come over to do some physicals on our admitted patients so they can go upstairs to the units. It's about one in the morning and he seems to be in no hurry to return to the AES. He sits down to chat with me and tells me a story about how they got a bunch of cops in the ER after the Million Man March in Harlem. The police were spraying mace into the crowd, but the wind blew it back in their faces and most of them had to seek medical attention. After a bit of back-and-forth banter, he yawns and stretches his arms.

As they go over his head, I see his plaid boxers peeking over the edge of his aqua scrubs, the hair from his umbilicus to his pubis exposed.

"Don't do that!" I shriek. "What are you trying to do to me?"

He looks confused, and I attempt to explain. "Those boxers, your scrubs, that happy trail. You're killing me!"

A huge grin spreads over his face. He is married; I have a boyfriend. But I have admitted to him that I am turned on by him, and he is pleased as punch.

He thinks he does it for me, and I'll have to let his assumption stand unchallenged. I don't have the heart to tell him it's his pants.

You Can't Do That

Even though we've started to peel away the layers of my sadism like an onion, my behavior is slow to change. Despite Mary's best efforts, one Monday afternoon in her office, I have a story to tell that suggests I still have a long way to go.

The previous night a prisoner had come in as a transfer from Columbia Presbyterian, after threatening the medical ER doc there. He'd been arrested for extortion, robbery, and assault, and taken to Columbia because of a large cut on his right hand incurred during the assault. A laceration needs to be sutured within nine hours usually, and since he had refused medical attention at Columbia—hence the threat to the ER doc—he was now working on twelve. I went to talk to him in the locked area, to see if I could schmooze him into having his hand looked at. I was ready for a really nasty, help-rejecting patient, but when he finally rolled in, he was actually calm and pleasant. He had no psychiatric history, denied all the usual symptoms like auditory hallucinations or suicidal ideation, and denied any substance abuse besides alcohol. When I asked how often he got into fights, he said, "Whenever I can," with a smirk.

He was initially friendly with me, complimenting me, acting sort of sexy and ultracasual. He let me examine his hand, and he accepted my recommendation to let the hand surgeons take a look. I figured we were good to go. I decided to medicate him with a mild anti-anxiety medicine so he would stay calmer for their exam. I knew the surgeons wouldn't put up with any attitude or ambivalence; they'd just write in the chart that the guy refused treatment and that'd be the end of it. (The surgeons hate to come down to the CPEP. They're just like everyone else that way.) After I spoke with the hand surgeon and got him to agree to come down, the patient changed his mind, and decided that he didn't want anyone to touch his hand.

I got really pissed off then. I argued with him for a while and got nowhere, and then I called him a pussy.

"You know what, sister? When I get out of these handcuffs, I'm gonna come back to this hospital and kick the shit out of you. That's what you need and I know it. I know where to find you, you fucking cunt."

"That's Doctor Cunt to you, you fucking weasel," I said as I stood in front of his locked wheelchair. "You're just chickenshit to have the surgeons sew your hand." I ridiculously believed I could double-dog dare him into having sutures. He was handcuffed to the chair, and as he tried to get out and lunge at me, I flinched and walked quickly into the nurses' station. As soon as I got in and shut the door, Chuck, the nurse in charge for the night, looked at me and grinned. "Oh, yeah, that was real professional."

Mary and I have talked a lot about my need for self-control. I am mortified to have to convey this story to her. It's a painful but necessary part of my therapy.

"Look, I know that it's never okay to talk to a patient like that. There's no excuse for acting like I did. I know it's horrible."

"Go on," she encourages.

I skillfully skirt the whole issue of sadism, but let her know I know it's there. "It's not just sadistic, it's masochistic. I could've gotten killed."

"I don't doubt that. But what do you think was going on?" Mary asks.

"One thing I've noticed: All of these guys that I do this with, they're all in cuffs. Lucy and I have talked about this. Give us a man in shackles and we try to push him around. We sort of get in his face and poke him in the chest—metaphorically, I mean. Or maybe literally. I never taunt anyone who's in hospital restraints. It's just the cuffs. Maybe it's something about his being an acknowledged dangerous person, like sticking my head in a lion's mouth? Did Lucy ever talk to you about this?"

"You know I can't answer that," Mary says.

"Oh yeah, of course I do," I assent. I can never forget that Lucy was

Mary's patient, but I do conveniently omit that she can't discuss any of their treatment. It's frustrating to me and probably to her, too. Mary could probably offer me some answers ahead of schedule, tidbits she's figured out in her work with Lucy, but she can't. I wonder if she gets bored hearing it all over again, groaning to herself, *Oh, please. Here we go again with the butch taunting of the prisoners.*

"Well, one thing that might be related to the cuffs is that these guys are the ones most visibly locked up. I know I have a big issue with having the keys to the unit. I'm the one who has the power and the freedom, and the patients are the ones who're locked in. I feel horrible about it, but I end up turning that off . . . doing a one-eighty. I turn my guilt into something else. Something mean.

"When I first started working in psychiatry, the keys, the patients being locked in, it really got to me. At Sinai, one of the hardest things for me in the beginning was leaving the patients on the ward over the weekends. I would walk out on Friday, locking the door behind me as I left, and all the patients would stay locked up all weekend long. I'd come back on Monday morning, after biking in the park, going to a movie, a concert, whatever, and there they'd be, as if nothing had changed: all of them on the ward just as I left them. Like reading a book, closing it for the night, and when I pick it up to read it later, all the characters would be right there waiting for me."

"And how does this translate into you feeling guilty?" she prods.

"Well, I guess it's really about freedom. How I have the freedom to run around the city, go Rollerblading, lie in the grass sunbathing in the park, and the patients are locked up all weekend long like caged animals. It doesn't seem fair." I pause, thinking about what I said. "So . . . the keys. Having the keys is a big deal. I have the means of coming and going, of leaving the ward. Oh, you'll love this: When I was a resident at Sinai, doing a rotation at the Bronx VA, this huge patient, who was kind of simple, but I had a real love for him—I called him Uncle Louie 'cause he reminded me of my great uncle—he tried to choke me at the door. He was trying to escape and I was trying to shut the door and lock it, and he choked me with my own keys. They were on this long necklace, made out of some heavy string, like a shoelace, along with my hospital ID."

"What happened?" she asks, the concern in her voice revealing a maternal, protective tone that I can't help but savor for a moment.

"The nurses and psych techs wrestled him off me. They heard me making this kind of choking, gurgling sound, and came running. As they pulled him off me, I remember feeling weakened, broken. I couldn't understand why nice old Uncle Louie would do that to me. I think I probably sank to the floor, my back against the door, guiltily watching the restraint and sedation that followed. That's how they did it, you know? There was no discussion or anything."

"Wow."

"Yeah, so, ever since then I don't wear keys around my neck, and I encourage the residents and medical students not to also. I keep my keys in my pocket. There are plenty of things a patient can use to hurt you, but the keys around my neck seemed terribly symbolic to me, right? It made me feel like I shouldn't be dangling them in front of everyone's faces, like the jailer with his jangling keys to the cells. Or the zookeeper."

"Well, the thing that seems interesting to me is that this is a major part of your job in the psych ER, though. Plenty of locked doors, different keys, security guards, prisoners, am I right?"

"Right. It's a locked unit. Actually, all the psych units I've ever worked on have been locked units. It's been an issue from the very beginning: who stays in, who's allowed to leave. I think I've always had guilt about being the one with the keys, the one who can leave. I have zookeeper guilt."

She's not laughing.

"But now, at my new job, it's more than that. Before, when I was a resident, I could blame it on the doctor in charge. Now, I'm in charge. I'm deciding who can go and who can't. I am the one locking these people in."

"And?"

"And . . . hello? I feel guilty! I hate the responsibility. I don't want to be the bad guy. You know what else, I never wear the white coat. It's too authoritative. It just feels wrong to me."

"Well, as far as the guilt goes, I think it's all in the way you frame it, Julie. If you're helping these people, if they're getting medicine, and the medical attention they need, doesn't that help to assuage the guilt?"

"It should, yes. But . . . so . . . why was I such a bitch to this guy? The thing that gets me, that I can't let go of, is that he said yes at first. I thought I'd won him over and he was going to play ball. Then, when I get everything organized, the surgeon's coming, the patient's medicated, he changes his mind. It was infuriating. I thought I had an alliance with the patient. We're on the same page. But why do I take it so personally when he changes his mind?"

"Do you think you felt betrayed, on some level?" suggests Mary.

"But how can I feel so betrayed by a man I don't even know? Who's a known criminal, probably a sociopath? There's a narcissistic element at play here too, don't you think? Like, I thought I was special, I could tame the lion that no one else could. And him changing his mind makes me look bad to the surgeons, like I can't control my patient."

"I have a feeling if this prisoner was waiting for a consult from an endocrinologist we wouldn't be having this conversation," Mary says astutely.

"You're all over it, Mary, as usual. I'll always have a thing for those guys. There's something about me prepping him for the surgeons, like I'm part of the surgical team. They don't want their time wasted, and I don't want to be seen as the one who dropped the ball. But the other important thing is that our interaction started out very casually, and flirty. You know that's something I do at my job a lot, I flirt. And it usually works. The guy thinks if we were at a bar instead of the ER, I'd probably give him my number, so he agrees to whatever I'm asking. But here, he was going to play it my way, and then he turned on me, somehow. It's almost like being rejected sexually, too, not just in a doctor-patient framework, y'know? It's like I got shot down. I think that's why I exploded so much more than usual."

"You think we need to talk more about that? That you flirt at work?" Mary asks.

"Yeah, we definitely do. I need to understand it better. I know it has something to do with blurring the boundaries, changing the roles of doctor and patient. I guess that's something else I do to even out the power imbalance. Like when I was a resident, and even when I first started at Bellevue, I used to sit on the floor with the patients and interview them there."

"Why on earth would you do that?"

"Same reason: to even things out. To show the patient I'm down with them, man! I'm on their level. I'm cool."

"So, how cool were you last night?"

"Touché. Not so much."

"Right."

It's getting near the end of the session. I can tell by the way her "right" hangs in the air. She's not starting a new thread for me to take up.

There is precious little instant gratification going on in this office. Becoming self-aware, making changes in behavior, these things take time. The knots may be loosening, but nothing will be untangled today.

I leave her office wordlessly.

The Letter

I arrive for my shift on Saturday night and check my mailbox, which typically houses junk mail from pharmaceutical companies or medical journals. Tonight a personal letter is in my slot, postmarked May 12 from Philadelphia. The address on the envelope is handwritten to me at Bellevue and includes the correct zip code, my full name, and two different ways to refer to my department: CPEP and Psych ER. Whoever wrote this clearly wanted it to reach me, but there is no return address. I assume it has come from a patient who spent some time here recently. It is a rare event to receive a thank-you note, but it does happen.

Inside the envelope is a condom wrapped in a blank piece of paper. The condom is enormous, the biggest I've ever seen. On another piece of paper, similarly folded into thirds, is a laser-printed note:

Julie Whore:

Take a dildo, this divine f.l. and fuck #1 your fucking cunt, #2 your stupid ass, #3 your fucking mouth, #4 your fucking tits & finish off by fucking your stinking pussie.

The coksman.

I bring it into the CPEP and show it to some of the residents and medical students, and we deduce the following: The guy's not much of a speller, and f.l. means French letter, a term I had never heard. One of the doctors mentions that Elvis sang about it once, and it referred to a condom. (Later, Jeremy explains that it was Elvis Costello. I had assumed it was The King.) How this particular condom has been made divine I don't even want to imagine.

On Monday morning, I bring the envelope and its enclosures to the NYPD, who give me a case number but don't want to read the letter or keep it for evidence. Perhaps I am naive to think that anyone would want to try to track down the sender, but I feel like it should be kept somewhere safe in case some sociopath comes after me. I give a Xeroxed copy to the head of hospital security at Bellevue the following Monday morning.

"If you find me chopped up in little pieces, maybe this will help you solve the puzzle," I joke. I then remember that, a few years back, a pregnant pathologist was strangled upstairs late at night by a homeless man who was living in the boiler room of the hospital. Maybe the head of security won't think my joke is that funny.

The day I got the letter, Jeremy had told me that he was worried about me at the hospital. It was a Saturday afternoon, and we were in Central Park when I ran into a schizophrenic I knew from my years at Mount Sinai. I couldn't remember his name fast enough, and so I squeezed his arm and said hello. He walked on for a few steps, turned around, and then shouted at me, "Little girl! This is my house! Just you remember that!" referring, I assumed, to the park itself, or maybe simply to the world outside the hospital.

"He's not usually so hostile," I explained to Jeremy. "He's probably just sick right now, probably off his meds."

This triggered a conversation about the hazards of my job. As if to drive the point home, it was when I went to work later that evening that I found the letter in my mailbox. The whole idea of it nauseated me, instructing me what to do to my own body with a phallus, like a sexual assault by proxy. Later that night in my call-room, I kept jumping up, listening and waiting, every time I heard the door to the suite click open down the hall.

The letter confirmed my suspicions: I had ticked somebody off, big-time. Despite my work with Mary, I continued to be confrontational in dangerous situations. Going up against big, scary guys persisted as one of my favorite pastimes, especially if I thought the patient was lying, pretending to be mentally ill. Discharging malingerers was a routine part of my job, and catching them at lying was easy. "You suck at lying," I would say derisively. "Why don't you try Beth Israel down the street. Maybe they'll fall for it." Sometimes, I'd even give them a few tips on how to make their story more effective. I'd pull them aside, conspiratorially, "Listen, just because I'm not buying what you're selling doesn't mean you can't find someone who will. Here's what you gotta do . . ." But other times, I was just an asshole, kicking them out of a warm place.

When I first started working at CPEP, the patients I would typically go after were arrested and handcuffed to a chair. I could piss them off as much as I dared, and they were like helpless little kittens: They couldn't really fight back. Somewhere along the way, though, I had gotten cocky. I forgot that the ones who weren't shackled could be just as dangerous as the ones who were. They wouldn't all take my castrating stance so quietly. Sooner or later I was going to take a pounding.

I had kicked out at least three fakers in the week preceding the letter. After I let a patient know he's leaving, I usually walk him to the door myself, bringing him back out in front of the hospital police to wait for his shoelaces. One man got right up in my face out there by the door, calling me a whore, screaming, "Fuck you!" and "Fuck your mother!" Maybe he sent the letter.

Another man had made up a story about how he had crossed Canal Street in Chinatown, walked into traffic in an effort to kill himself, but then a car stopped and a man got out to "save his life" and brought him to Bellevue. The Good Samaritan scenario in New York City is always a hard sell with me. Over multiple interviews, this man changed the car to a van, and then a city bus. He told the medical student and resident who interviewed him that his brother had committed suicide two weeks ago and he went to the funeral, even though he mentioned he'd just gotten out of jail the day before. (If I had a nickel for every dead person I've spoken to on the phone, I'd have a dollar thirty-five by now.) He floundered on dates and locations, telling me he had crossed the street north to south, later telling me south to north. I like to play detective with the lying patients, and when I catch them in their lies, I usually call them on it. I've seen one too many episodes of *NYPD Blue*, I think.

The weekend before I received the letter, I had kicked out a lying patient who was from Philadelphia, and he swore he would "come back to hunt me down." The postmark is from Philadelphia. Maybe the letter's from him.

I decide to compile a list of likely patients by combing through the discharge records from the past few weekends. I'll give the list to hospital security and to NYPD. A detective assigned to the case comes by my apartment to speak to me and leaves his card under my door, since I'm not home. When I ask the doorman about it, he has no recollection of letting the man in.

I explain why he should be extra-cautious about anyone who says he is there to see me.

Swimming with Sharks

It begins as a day unlike any other: nine o'clock, Wednesday morning, May 20, 1998, and I'm shot full of drugs. Lying on a stretcher, I am mildly amused at the television show I'm watching: It is my colon, bloodred and slick with mucus.

"Fabulous," gushes my doctor. I nod my head in agreement. It is my first colonoscopy, surprisingly painless. Maybe it's just the Demerol and Valium talking, but I am pleasantly conversant throughout the procedure. Afterwards, it takes several hours to come down from my high. As I walk back to my apartment, I delight at my surroundings. It is a beautiful spring day, unseasonably warm. The trees are flowering on Park Avenue, and there are tulips and daffodils in the gardens in front of the high rises.

I am working tonight, subbing in for my best pal Lucy, and I decide—as I glide home, stoned—to walk to the hospital, seventy blocks south. After working at Bellevue for two years, it will be my first time walking there. (Over my nine years there, I will never walk to work again.)

I arrive for rounds a few minutes late, glistening with sweat. Lucy pulls me aside after sign-out and tells me in the hallway that it's official: She's been made Director of CPEP. Dr. Lear is leaving, and he has picked her to be his replacement. I am thrilled for her. For us.

"Are you sure I can't convince you to work weekdays with me?" Lucy asks. "You could be my assistant director. We'd be a hell of a team."

"I know we would, and I would so love to be your right-hand man, dudette. But I've gotten very used to my weeks off. I love flying solo on the weekends; you know that. I just can't give up this schedule. Even for you."

"I know you can't. I probably wouldn't do it if I were you," she smiles. She then asks me what I think about Daniel. "You know him from Sinai, right? I'm thinking about pulling him from 18 North to work at CPEP. You think it's a góod idea? Daniel down here to be the assistant director?"

"Well, he'd certainly be an improvement over the one we have now. He'll be fine . . . sure," I say, trying to convince myself as I sell Lucy. It's hard to imagine working side by side with Daniel again after Sinai. I'm not sure how I feel about it exactly, but I don't share my indecision with Lucy. I don't want to pull the focus away from her promotion. She's been told to keep it quiet for a while, mostly out of respect for the current A.D. who thought the job would be his, so I spend the first part of my shift feeling like the cat who ate the canary. I know staff morale will skyrocket once everyone hears the news—everyone loves the ballsy and charismatic Lucy.

The CPEP gets busier as the afternoon wears on. I usually start my shift a bit later when I work the weekends: Working for Lucy on a Wednesday means coming in at four instead of seven. I'm happy to do her this favor, but it occurs to me soon after she leaves that it's going to be a long night.

The skies darken early; a hard rain is imminent. The EMS cases start pouring in. I hear Rita, behind her desk, on the phone talking to her son, "No, seriously, it's hailing now?!"

The last time I was in a May hailstorm was in a rental car in the middle of wide-open "Color Country" in Utah. The hail pounded on the roof, and Jeremy and I were absolutely panicked that a tornado would come barreling through the prairie and take the car up into its funnel. Rita says "hail," I think *panic*.

The nondetainable area is filling up, and the night has a weird vibe to it. It feels like being on a ship that is taking in water from all sides. Not only is one ambulance case after another coming in, but I am getting a lot of calls from other hospitals. Everyone else is full, the rest of the city is jam-packed with psych cases, but for some reason Bellevue has scads of empty beds—the only beds in the city. So I am accepting transfers from other hospitals, which always pisses off the nurses, adding to everyone's workload. I am obligated to take the psychotic prisoner referrals, but I also accept a couple of homeless guys with no insurance, knowing full well no other hospital will accept these patients since they can't pay for services.

And now, to make matters worse, the ER is dumping wrist slits on me: two in a row, back-to-back transfers, both drunk at the time they cut their wrists, and both sober now. One had lethal intent—he really was hoping the cuts would be deep enough for him to bleed to death, so he gets admitted upstairs to an inpatient psych bed. The other is a drunk "hitting bottom," as they say, with superficial cuts requiring no sutures. We confirm with him that this is a "cry for help," and he is admitted to a detox bed.

There are so many patients on triage that not only the moonlighters—three hired hands to help out with the evening overflow—but also the medical students are having to see cases individually. "Divide and conquer!" I encourage them, even though the medical students typically work in pairs or shadow the moonlighters.

It's raining like crazy out there; the lightning strobes against the EOU windows. The resident on-call presents a new case to me, and as we discuss it, I sense that her new patient is malingering. He gave conflicting stories to the triage nurse and the resident, and he's keeping a very low profile in the ER, slouching down underneath a yellow hooded sweatshirt like he's hiding out. I ask the resident to reinterview the patient, and now he's saying anything he can think of to be admitted, upping the ante with each interview, but he's having trouble keeping his story straight. I go out to speak with him after I notice that he's given the clerk a home address that's very near my own, a nice block on the Upper East side. I'm curious about his living in my neighborhood, and when I ask him where the block is, he tells me it's between Second and Third, though the address he gave the clerk is between Park and Madison. I question him about this, and he then "admits" it is his wife's address and that they are separated.

"And you're confused about what block she lives on since the separation?" I jab. He looks at me quizzically, angrily, and I get up to leave, quitting while I'm ahead.

When the resident and I rehash the case in the nurses' station, we decide that the patient is "F.O.S." (full of shit) and needs to leave. He isn't mentally ill; he's clearly faking it in order to gain admission to the hospital. We're pretty sure he's a sociopath; we sometimes call them sharks. Guys like this enjoy their time in the hospital, easier than the streets or shelters, and certainly more cushy than jail time, which is where most sharks end up. It's my job to make sure that sociopaths don't get into Bellevue. Not only do they take up a bed that could be better utilized, but they also make the hospital a more dangerous place. Sharks have a tendency toward violence and they prey on the weak—in this case, the vulnerable psychiatric patients.

As always, I am eager to kick out a malingerer, excising him like a malignant tumor. As I go out to talk to him, a moonlighting doctor suggests that I take someone with me, that maybe this patient is dangerous. Walking out of the nurses' station, I say brazenly, "I've been here two years and haven't gotten tagged yet. Maybe I'm due."

I walk over to the man in the yellow sweatshirt, and he responds to my inquiries very quietly. So quietly, in fact, that I need to lean in toward him so that I can hear his responses.

"Mr. Brown, we're having a little problem regarding your patient information. It's just not adding up," I begin.

"So?"

"So, some of the doctors here think that you may be feigning your illness."

"Feigning?" he asks.

"Faking," I explain.

And then it comes. A huge fist flies into my face, and as I hear the smack, I see a flash of bright white light. I stagger backwards from the force of the blow. Eleanor, the largest female psych tech we have, is on him in a heartbeat, tackling him to the ground, while I take another step back, and then another, stunned.

"I got him, Doc," Eleanor calls to me proudly as I scurry back to the nurses' station.

"I want to press charges, Eleanor!" I shout back to her. The hospital police have already come to help out, reminding me that this is an option, and I want them to take him away. Rocky is there, front and center, acting professionally, not making a big deal of the irony that I can't help but notice. The guy I almost got fired is now the cop who'll arrest my shark.

I sit down for a minute, shaky, talking nervously, trying to make light of the whole scene, and the next thing I know one of the medical ER doctors has run over to check me out. It's a good friend of Lucy's, another lesbian with a down-home drawl I feel a special connection to, and I'm glad she's on duty tonight. She helps me feel I'm in capable, caring hands as she masterfully palpates the cheekbones under my eyes to feel for a fracture, and recommends I get a skull X-ray just to be sure. I sit in the radiology suite like a patient, with a rubber glove filled with ice pressed against the bruise beginning to form on my cheek, and I try not to cry.

When the buzz has died down in CPEP, and my facial series has been cleared by the radiologist, I lie low in the nurses' station, not willing to go home and abandon my shift, but also not fully willing to reengage with the patients or the paperwork.

Later Rocky comes by to tell me that Mr. Brown has been arrested and taken to the thirteenth precinct. He makes a point of relating to me the opening sentence on the arrest paperwork. Rocky has quoted him word for word, "I wanted to hit the doctor. I hope I got her good."

I imagine it will be hard to plead innocent with a statement like that. When I speak to the assistant district attorney later in the week, I learn that the man has over twenty "priors." They don't even need me to come down to testify. I fax over some short forms and the deed is done. He will spend the next four months at Rikers.

Jeremy figures that this guy needed to be off the streets so badly, if he couldn't be admitted to the hospital, he'd do his time in jail instead. Otherwise, why be so bold about punching me, setting me up with his quiet voice, confessing to it immediately? Or is it just that he is a bad guy? Maybe he's simply a violent man who doesn't care what the consequences are, he just wanted to "get me good."

What I can't stop wondering is, Did he get me good enough? Might he come looking for me when he gets out of Rikers to get me again?

Save Me

On Monday, I play a little game with Mary to see if she can see the bruise on my face. "Notice anything different about me?"

"Did you get your hair cut?" she asks, confused.

"Not exactly. Look at my cheek."

"Ooh, how'd you get that?" she asks, getting up off her chair to examine my bruise.

"Funny story," I begin, but of course, just hearing myself try to make a joke of it, I begin to cry. I cover my face with my hands to hide the ugly grimaces that typically accompany my tears.

"What happened?" she asks, so caring and concerned, so loving and open and able. She is standing right in front of me, not quite sitting back down in her chair, although I imagine she wishes she'd never gotten up.

Part of me wants her to hold me, and to comfort me. The more grown-up part, the psychiatrist in me, knows that this would be inappropriate, and that I need to soldier on, to talk about it so we can do our work.

"I got punched in the face by a patient."

She sits down in her chair and waits. She's not going to say a word until I completely unload. I could never be this patient with a patient. She has so much to teach me about being a good therapist. I need to remember to wait while I listen.

"I called him on his shit and he punched me. He whispered real quiet so I had to lean in to hear him and then he popped me, hard, right in my face. Have you ever been punched?" I ask, rhetorically. No self-respecting shrink would answer that, I imagine.

"No, I haven't," she answers calmly.

"I hadn't either. It's really interesting, the physics of it. It's like a cartoon caption. You know, the ones that say BLAM! There's a big white jagged disc that accompanies the fist, that spins off of the impact. The energy of a fist and a face, when they collide, it creates a separate thing. It's got heat. It vibrates. It actually pushed me backwards."

"I think maybe you need to get beyond the interesting physics of the collision here, Julie. Can you tell me why this happened?" Mary makes it clear that I'm wasting valuable time.

"He was a malingerer. He was lying about his address and I caught him on it. I confronted him, told him I thought he was lying, and he punched me."

"Is there more?" she asks simply.

"I'm sure he thought I was being a smug asshole."

"And you think?"

"That he was probably right. I couldn't wait to call him on it. Jeremy says it was emasculating. And that is obviously not therapeutic. He says I'm not helping these patients. Whatever is going on with them, whether they're lying or telling the truth, the bottom line is they're coming to me as a physician for assistance and then leaving empty-handed. I'm leaving them hanging. Dissatisfied. Only worse than that. They're insulted."

"It's probably humiliating enough for them to be in the position of approaching the Bellevue psych ER asking for assistance. You don't need to add to their shame."

"So why did I do that? I think I get caught up in the cat and mouse of it. I get excited that I've figured out their game. I'm on to them and I want them to know they're not getting anything past me. But that's not what it should be about, right?"

"Right."

While I'm talking, I'm also reviewing: First she hears about the razor man, then the transfer from Columbia. Last week I told her about the letter from Philly. This week I tell her about getting punched in the face. She must be feeling she's got her work cut out for her. I hate that, feeling like a problem patient. Maybe she can't fix me? Or worse, it's too hard and she can't be bothered.

"And then, the morning after I got punched, I came home and couldn't leave the apartment again. I was feeling really twitchy. I couldn't do my errands, but I also couldn't nap. I couldn't stop my brain. I finally left the house in the evening to meet Jeremy for a movie. When I went down the subway stairs, I kept flinching if anyone got too close to me. I had an increased startle response just like post-traumatic patients do. And then, during the movie, I couldn't concentrate on the plot. I just kept seeing his fist coming into my face. The image intruded onto my mind's eye, and I'd flinch every time."

"Increased startle response, intrusive recollections. Classic PTSD symptoms," says Mary.

"Exactly. It was actually fascinating for me to experience them, and to know that this is what patients really do go through after a trauma. I feel like I'll be better able to warn people about potential symptoms after an assault having gone through it."

"Great, Julie," she groans. "Can we get to work here?"

"Yeah, I know. My behavior is totally humiliating and emasculating, which is therefore provocative and confrontational. Okay? I get it."

"And?" Mary has not heard what she wants just yet.

"I have got to learn to rein myself in."

"Bingo. You. Yourself. No one is going to do this for you, Julie. You can't be all gas and no brake."

As Mary points out, I could've gotten hurt much worse than I did. I'm lucky *he* reined himself in with just one exacting punch. There was a resident at Mount Sinai who was assaulted by a patient and he repeatedly slammed her head against the floor. She was never the same again. I still remember the stunned look in her eyes when I'd talk to her. It lasted for weeks after it happened.

I'm lucky it wasn't worse.

Run for Your Life

After I get punched in the face, it's pretty much business as usual for the next few weekends, except for one thing: I have become a bit gun-shy, like a skittish rabbit, quickly scurrying away at the first sign of trouble.

At sign-out I hear about a fifty-seven-year-old homeless man who came in by ambulance, grossly psychotic and disorganized. He's coming off a seven-year stint in prison for homicide after beating a man to death with his bare hands, instead of using a gun like a civilized criminal. As usual, the Department of Corrections didn't come up with any sort of game plan for how a man like this, with a psychotic illness and a violent past, is supposed to fend for himself in the outside world upon release. A lot of these prisoners quickly end up at Bellevue where we try to put something together for them—a doctor who can treat them on an ongoing basis and a place to sleep.

I go to find my new patient in the observation room across from the nurses' station. He has been placed on Hold status during the shift prior to mine, and he needs to be reevaluated for a potential admission. There are several patients in the observation room, all of them sleeping. I approach a patient who is curled up on a stretcher with his back turned to me, and I say, "Excuse me, sir, are you Mr. Taylor or Mr. Richards?"

There is no reply.

"Okay, now, I don't know if you're sleeping or just not talking, so I'm just going to take a look at your arm band here." I slide the sheet off his clothed body to get a look at his right wrist.

He swings around, growls, "Don't touch me!" and lunges toward me.

As fast as I can, I run out of the room and into the nurses' station, locking the door behind me. I am quaking.

The nurses medicate him while I read his chart. Probably shoulda done this first. What would've been nice to know at sign-out is that the day before, he had required restraints and medication after threatening to beat up the staff and to rape any women in the area. He had also advised a female attending to "Wipe out your pussy."

If I'd known this ahead of time, his explosion of unpredictable behavior wouldn't have caught me so off guard. He's lying in wait with his back to me one minute, awake and silent, and the next he's pouncing like a tiger. But would I really have gotten all that from reading the chart?

I am now timid, to say the least, about seeing dangerous patients. I appreciate the nurses' not giving me a hard time about it. I suppose that anyone would've backed away in that situation, but running into the nurses' station and locking the door? I'm not so sure. It feels different now, like the stakes are higher; all of a sudden, pain is a real possibility, so it's appropriate to be cautious. But I can't let my fear stand in the way of being their doctor.

Then there is the issue of confronting patients who are lying and need to leave. I need to put into practice what I have been learning in my work with Mary.

Be kind. Be therapeutic. Be understanding. Don't be a complete bitch.

Even the lying patients are still coming to the hospital because they are in need. Don't send them away empty-handed.

I probably should've been reminded of these simple things earlier in the game. Stay safe, be gentle, deferential even. My tough-guy confrontational thing is so over.

It starts to come as second nature after a while, and as the weeks go by, I comfortably ease into my new role as Florence Nightingale.

And then things start to get weird.

About a month after the assault, and for the next several weekends, my pager goes off in the middle of the night. This is extremely unusual;

I never get paged. If anyone wants to find me, they call the CPEP. But now, at three or four in the morning, weekend after weekend, I wake to the shrill sound of my beeper. I press the button that backlights the numbers. It is always the same, or nearly the same: a variation on a theme. 69696969. Sometimes only a single 69.

Someone is fucking with me.

Turn the Page

The mysterious stalker paging continues for nearly a month. I'm getting used to my beeper having multiple 696969s displayed in its memory. They come only on the weekends when I am at the hospital, usually while I'm sleeping in my office, and never when I'm at home or earlier in the day. It's as if someone is telling me they know my schedule: when I'm at CPEP, and when I go to bed.

There is something eerie about getting paged like this. It is intimate, intrusive, and taunting. I am frightened, staring into the darkness, alone in my call-room at three in the morning, contemplating horror-movie scenarios. Who the hell is doing this? Am I supposed to think it's funny? Could they possibly be thinking it's sexy and I should be turned on or flattered? Is it Jude or Paul or one of the other AES attendings I flirt with?

Or is it someone trying to scare me?

Because I am not turned on. I am scared.

I start watching my back as I walk around the hospital. I roam the deserted hallways afraid I will bump into a rapist or a barrage of fists as I round the corners. Remembering the episodes on *ER* where the attending Mark Green gets beaten up in the bathroom and ends up abusing painkillers, I start using the bathroom in the nurses' station instead of the more secluded one near my office on the other side of the hall.

I feel especially vulnerable when I park my car in the garage coming to work in the evening. The fluorescent bulbs cast an ocher tint on the concrete and steel, and I run up the flight in the echoing stairwells, afraid to spend more than a moment in the desolate structure. I am relieved as I leave the garage and enter First Avenue, comforted by the sight of the homeless men and drunks that hang out around the front entrance, some of whom I know by name. Rocky's patrolling the front walk, and I flash him a smile, truly glad to see him.

Fire in the Hole

It's the usual Thursday morning staff meeting, July 1998, followed by the usual smaller faculty meeting. We're spending way too much time talking about a proposed crisis residence—temporary housing with significant mental health support services. Anywhere besides a shelter to send a mentally ill person is inherently a good thing, so we all agree that this is needed. What we can't seem to agree upon is the structure of the research project to prove its worth. If this is going to slow down the creation of a crisis residence, I'm going to need my own mental health support services. The bureaucracy of New York City is slowly driving me insane. At least it's taking my mind off the stalker situation.

Disgusted, I get up to use the bathroom attached to the conference room, where the water in the bowl is perpetually brown, and I assume my colleagues can hear my every tinkle. A set of alarm bells begins to ring as I sit on the bowl. Three sets of seven blasts repeat at regular intervals. I can hear the doctors outside the door wondering aloud what the code means. All fire alarms at Bellevue are coded; a series of 7, then 1, then 4 (like the old Lemmon 714 Quaalude) signifies a fire in the CPEP. No one knows what 7-7-7 means, but I do.

"INTERNAL/EXTERNAL DISASTER!!!" I have to yell above the sound of the toilet flushing.

I know this because at the interminable staff meeting a half hour earlier, I was reading a poster while the head nurse droned on. The poster, on the wall above the crash cart, deciphers all the bell codes, and specifically mentions this disaster code.

The meeting breaks up as the bells continue to sound, and everyone seems stymied as to what's going on. I call Jeremy and ask him to turn on the news to find out what disaster has befallen the city, and to page me if he hears anything.

Pam, one of the other attendings, calls the AES to see if they know anything, and is told that they now have twenty-six cases of anthrax in their ER. This is three years before anthrax has become a household word, and I have to look up the treatment in my infectious disease handbook. I immediately dial a pharmacy near Jeremy's apartment to phone in a prescription for Cipro, enough for both of us, as I scream to the other doctors that anthrax is treatable; it's a bacteria. Pam counters that she's pretty sure it is immediately lethal, and there is no treatment. I repeat, in my most sure and doctorly tone, that it is treatable with antibiotics, as I am put on hold at the SoHo pharmacy. I fantasize there will be a run on Cipro as the news breaks, and I need to get through before the other people in the city learn what has happened.

Another doctor, who's called his wife, says there's nothing on CNN. "They probably don't want to start a panic," I surmise, projecting my inner state onto the network executives. I call Jeremy back and tell him calmly that there are twenty-six cases of anthrax in the ER, and I have called in a prescription for prophylaxis for both of us, and when it is safe to go outside, he should pick up the pills at his corner drugstore.

"When it's safe to go outside?" he asks, his voice tremulous. He sounds scared and I wish that he weren't.

"I'll call you back when I know more," I say, as a way of saying good-bye but not leaving him entirely.

Pam and I go to the AES to investigate. As we walk over, I find myself worried that perhaps we shouldn't be around people with anthrax. "Is it contagious?" I ask.

"I don't think it's spread by person-to-person contact," she answers. This from the gal who says it's immediately lethal and untreatable, and yet I opt to take her guess as fact. We go through a set of double doors where a hospital policewoman is sitting.

"Is it okay to pass through here?" I ask, thinking the AES may be quarantined.

She shrugs her shoulders in typical infuriating Bellevue fashion—
don't ask me, I just work here. We burst through the doors of the medical ER expecting a scene of chaos and fear: police, reporters, and extra
staff pouring in due to the disaster alarms. What we find is a quiet and
calm scene, no more people than usual, perhaps even fewer. Everyone
is going about their business. In the corner, the Director of the AES is
surrounded by people in suits, each one carrying a piece of typewritten
paper, its heading: Anthrax Disaster Drill.

I am deflated, angry that no one told us ahead of time about the drill.
Who answered the phone and reported twenty-six cases of anthrax to
a CPEP doctor? Were they instructed to say this? Don't they know how
easily something like this can go from rumor to fact to widespread panic?
I call Jeremy back to tell him it's a false alarm, but he's already called his
two sisters who live in the city, fearing that they've been caught outside
when the biological warfare was launched. I apologize strenuously, feeling sheepish, but we decide to get the prescription filled anyway.

If Bellevue is having a drill, we may as well be prepared for the real
thing.

Skeletons

I have told no one about the paging aside from Jeremy and Mary. I vacillate between thinking it is a harmless prank and feeling as though I am being spied upon and haunted. I'm not sure if the paging is connected to the "Julie whore" letter or not. I don't know how many people have it in for me, though my love of efficiency hopes it's only one.

And then one night, a new phone number glows from my pager, the beeping startling me out of sleep: 561-6969.

This is a clue. 561 is the old Bellevue exchange from the mid-nineties when I started working; it changed to 562 after a year or two. It must be coming from someone at the hospital. But why the old exchange? Is it a longtime employee? Maybe it's someone who used to work at Bellevue but doesn't anymore?

Working alone, I play the sleuth. The 561 smells like a slipup. The hidden harasser is giving himself away.

I skim through my mental Rolodex, recalling past Bellevue employees. CPEP has a pretty high turnover: Images of people who have come and gone flip like pages of a photo album in my mind. It could've been anyone: the guy who wheels patients to X-ray, one of the coffee shop waiters. Anyone.

I rack my brains as I stroll down memory lane, and then . . . I remember.

I inhale sharply, putting my hand to my open mouth. I know. And I *know* I know.

On the night of the FDR rape case, I received a transfer from another city hospital. I hadn't been called ahead of time about the patient, but someone had sent him anyway, putting my name as the accepting doctor on the transfer form. The name of the doctor sending the patient was Martin, the moonlighter who had called Dr. Lear at home on Christmas day. The moonlighter who thinks he was fired because of me.

When I saw his name, I only thought, *Oh, I guess he got a job somewhere else after all.* It's kind of an asshole thing to do, send a patient without permission, but I didn't think too much of it beyond that. He probably remembered I work there on the weekends, so he put my name down. But I guess this must have stirred up some bad memories for him.

This is just a little too disturbing for me to wrap my head around. And is it just the paging or did he send that sick letter too?

I decide I'm done sleuthing; I need a real detective to take over, but I don't call the cops. I ask my pal, the head of the hospital police, if he can track down Martin at the other hospital. Is there any way he can get the HP there to figure out if he is the one who has been paging me?

They do, and he is.

The HP's review of the phone records from the psych ER where he works reveals that he's been calling my pager. They think the letter's from him, too. Martin has a sister in Philadelphia, which could explain the postmark on the envelope.

Okay, so, we have my stalker, and it's not a psych patient. It's another psychiatrist. The huge condom, that psychopathic letter, the months of paging, they all came from a shrink. A weekend CPEP attending, just like me. Doctor, heal thyself, man!

I call a colleague who works upstairs on the prison ward, a specialist in forensic psychiatry, to ask his advice. He knows scary sociopathic patients inside and out, and I pick his brain for guidance. Should I press charges? Should I let Martin know I figured it out, that I'm on to him? Would it be dangerous to confront him?

He recommends that I let it go. "In no way should you confront him. Given the personality structure of someone who would do this, any confrontation could inflame him."

Dude, where were you when I started this job?

Martin's hospital administration does confront him, though. They let him know that they have seen the phone records, and no more is said. Luckily, it is enough. The paging stops, but I am nervous. He must know that I know it's him. What if he tries to silence me?

It is a Wednesday night, shortly after the stalker mystery is solved, when I receive a frightening phone call. In my own bed at home at 2:30 in the morning, I listen to a recorded voice informing me that prisoner number 141021267 is being released at two p.m. the following day. It takes a moment for me to understand why I am getting this, an automated call from Rikers. Why am I being informed about a prisoner's release?

But by the time I put the receiver down, I get it. Mr. Brown, the man I put into prison for four months after he punched me out of my smarmy attitude, will be free to exact his revenge, and he knows where to find me.

It's pretty tricky to fall back asleep after a phone call like that.

Great. Now I have to watch my back twice as much. I don't know if an enraged, humiliated Martin is finally coming to sexually assault me in person, upgrading from the proxy method, or if the man I sent to Rikers will hunt me down to finish the job he had barely begun.

I start asking for a police escort to walk me to my car after work.

Mary is proud that I am asking for assistance in an appropriate way, but my father scoffs when I mention it. He asks, "Isn't there a self-defense class you can take or something?"

I have officially lost my mojo, and my father sounds as ashamed as he makes me feel. Even though I've been in therapy long enough to know better, he can still push my buttons, making me feel like that little kindergartner who had to learn not to ask for help.

Afraid to walk the halls alone, I stop leaving the ER during my shifts. I bring my dinner from home so I don't have to go to the coffee shop. Again I tell the doorman at my building to be extra-suspicious of anyone looking for me. I start to lift more weights at the gym and sign up for a kickboxing class.

I also stop carrying my pager. It doesn't happen all at once. First, I don't replace the dead battery; I keep forgetting. Then finally, I convince myself I don't really need to carry a beeper, and I stick it in my desk drawer.

If I dare leave the CPEP, I tell the nurses where I'll be: the AES, my call-room, the coffee shop. I give Jeremy the CPEP phone number. He was the only one who ever really paged me much, besides Martin.

Many Rivers to Cross

"I found a lump."

Lucy is calling me on a Saturday night from East Hampton. I'm at the CPEP in the nurses' station, with my feet up on the desk, signing charts.

"Where?" I ask. I put down my feet.

"It's in my neck."

I pause. *Careful what you say here.* "It's probably just a swollen lymph node," I offer.

"Of course it's a swollen lymph node, you idiot. I think my cancer's back."

"But it could just be a swollen node because you're sick. There's tons of reasons. Do you have a sore throat? A cold? Anything?" I am grasping at straws I'm sure she's already rifled through.

"Nope. Nothing," she says.

I don't want this to be happening. Not now. It's crazy for this to happen now, after her cancer's been gone so long. And also, not now that Sadie is pregnant. After Lucy and Sadie got settled in their newfound stability as a couple and as home owners, they took the ultimate leap of faith in each other, and in life itself. They decided to have a child together, choosing a sperm donor out of a book. I remember Lucy telling me about it, tickled because not only is the donor a tall, blond, blue-eyed and brilliant scientist, but he wrote in his profile that he loved Gorgonzola cheese and basset hounds. Sadie is carrying the child;

Lucy wasn't allowed to because of her history of breast cancer. Even though it was nearly five years ago, the fertility docs felt it was too risky. I remember thinking at the time that they were over-erring on the side of caution.

"Lucy, you're five years clean already, right? Why are you assuming the worst? It could be absolutely nothing." Our roles are preassigned. I will wear the rose-colored glasses while she looks through the glass darkly. Except that on the inside, I am fast-forwarding to a grim ending, yet completely unable to allow myself to discuss the possibility.

Lucy, however, is resigned to what will be and does not pretend otherwise. "Why not? Why not get completely freaked out? I have one swollen lymph node on one side of my neck. If it were on both sides, I'd say maybe you're right, maybe I have a sore throat or a cold and I somehow don't even know it. But it's on one side of my neck and we both know what that means. My cancer's back and I'm going to die. It was really just a matter of time. Five years clean. Turns out it doesn't mean a fucking thing."

We go back and forth a little more, the charade on a seesaw. I have a feeling she's right, and maybe she senses this, but I feel like I have to balance out her realistic assessment with my hopeful illusions, so I keep telling her not to worry and it's going to turn out to be nothing.

I need to get back to work and tell her so. I hang up the phone, dazed. I try not to worry about losing my friend and mentor, my hero, to breast cancer. Five years clean. Time to get on with your life. You got a big promotion? Buy a house, have a kid, celebrate! Oops, not so fast . . .

I need to think about all of this later. I've got a job to do and she hasn't even seen her oncologist yet.

There's no point in worrying about all of this now.

It's not going to change anything.

I'll Cry Instead

I am with Jeremy at Lucy's house in East Hampton, the summer of 1998, when she calls me from the city with the news: the lump in her neck is from her breast cancer. Her oncologist did a biopsy and a CT scan. The breast cancer has metastasized to her brain.

Just when it seems that she has it all, the pregnant wife, the house in the Hamptons, the director's position at CPEP, it all comes crashing down. Somebody up there has an exquisite sense of timing, if you ask me.

"Are you scared?" I ask her. I feel like the twelve-year-old girl from Kansas again, and as usual, when it comes to Lucy, I don't know what to say.

"Hell no! I'm not scared, I'm pissed!"

She sounds it, too. She already did her time, fought the fight. Why should she have to go through it all again?

"I love you," I say. It is the first time I have told her, and it is long overdue.

"I know you do, Jules. I love you too."

"I'm sorry this is happening to you," I say meekly. I hang up the phone and cry in Jeremy's arms. Maybe she's not scared, but I am. I'm scared for her, and I'm scared for me. I've never gone through this with someone. Dying. I know she has an epic struggle ahead of her, and even though she won the battle before, I'm afraid, ultimately, she is going to lose this war.

I have no clue how I can help her, how I can make this better. What can I give to her, to support her as she undergoes chemo, radiation, maybe more surgery? And how is Sadie, in her second trimester now, going to deal with this?

When I try to talk to Mary about it, we hit a touchy area. Because Lucy was Mary's patient, protocol dictates that my therapist become tight-lipped when I bring her up. Lucy is no longer seeing Mary, though I think, given the new circumstance, she should. I think Mary can help her through this, can offer more psychological support than I possibly could. I want Mary to be Lucy's therapist again, and I tell her so.

"You know that's between me and Lucy," chides Mary. "Why is it so important to you that she be back in therapy now?"

Always with the questions. Every good therapist asks instead of answers. We are taught to deflect certain questions with reflected queries, tossing it right back into your lap. For instance, if a patient asks, "How old are you?" a well-trained therapist should find out the patient's fantasies and wishes, such as "How old do you think I am?" meaning: How old do you want me to be? Any variation on "Why do you want to know that? How would that help you?" would be an appropriate answer in a shrink's office, but not in the outside world.

When I was in my residency, training to be a questioning psychiatrist, we used to play a game I called "shrink ping-pong." Whoever can't think up a question to lob back at the other doctor loses. "How are you feeling today?" "What would be important to know about that?" "Why do you feel the need to know why I'm asking?" It can go on endlessly. Kind of like the average psychotherapy session when you are skirting around the big issues, like, "I'm afraid my friend is going to die and I have no way to stop it, and I have no real means of helping her."

Lucy goes through weeks of radiation to shrink her brain tumors. She doesn't want anyone at work to know where her recurrence is, afraid they'll assume she has neurological or psychiatric symptoms and therefore can't pull her weight in the CPEP. They know something is up, but they are low on details. I watch her like a hawk, afraid she'll give herself away. I make her change her outgoing message in her office because she slurred a word. She makes fun of me for worrying so much about how she appears to others, but I want to protect her. She re-records her outgoing message to appease me, but soon it is obvious to everyone that she is sick. She loses her hair and starts to wear scarves to work, and then makeup. She's never worn makeup to work since I've known her, but now, because she is sicker, thinner, and bald, she feels it's best to put on a happy, colorful face.

HBO has been shooting a documentary about Bellevue's CPEP. The director, Mary Ann DeLeo, and the producer, Sarah Teale, spend weeks on end taping everyone going about their jobs. When I sign out on Monday mornings, the camera is right in my face, or else it is in Lucy's face. DeLeo is queen of the ultra close-up. Lucy and I joke that you can't turn around too fast or you'll get bonked by the lens. We try to keep up our witty banter when the camera is rolling, but it feels staged and stale. I wish the magic between us could be captured and aired for all to see. I love signing out to Lucy, seeing her agree with my diagnoses and treatment plans, laughing at my jokes. When she speaks up to add something, it is inevitably germane and wise. Will the HBO audience appreciate that?

Lucy refuses to see Mary Ann and Sarah while she is out sick. They want the cameras to follow her wherever she is, at home, at the on-cologist's. What they don't realize is that Lucy needs brain surgery to remove the tumors. They ask me to talk to her but I won't. I know Lucy won't budge on this one.

Halloween falls on a Saturday night and I decide to dress up for work. I find a blue dress, matching beret, and my old volleyball knee pads. I smear white toothpaste on the dress: Monica Lewinsky. I decide to visit Lucy on my way to work to show her my getup, and hopefully to cheer her up. I make sure to apply some red lipstick before I enter her apartment, so she can get the whole look. I never wear makeup to work, but tonight I have eye shadow and blush to complete the ensemble.

Lucy is home with Sadie, who is due any day now, watching basket-ball, sitting on her couch, bald—no scarf, no wig. They both get out of my outfit, and I walk back to my car, glad I made her. When I get to CPEP, Mary Ann is there. She films me and I show her the accessories to the costume: my cigar, an

Walt Whitman's *Leaves of Grass* I am carrying. (The ultimate betrayal, as far as I'm concerned, is that Bill shared the same book of poems with Hillary and Monica.)

Again, Mary Ann asks about Lucy. She wants to know how she is and when she'll be back. The star has been off the set for a while, and the director is anxious for her return. I let Mary Ann know that Lucy is doing better, I just saw her at her apartment, and that she should be back at work pretty soon.

Later, when I watch the final cut of the documentary, I notice how awkward Lucy seems as Mary Ann follows her out the door from CPEP one day. Lucy is leaving early to go see her oncologist.

"The doctor goes to see the doctor," Lucy muses, as the camera follows her down the hallway. Her hair is scattered in every direction of the compass, letting shards of light through to the camera. "The big C," Lucy jokes.

It is anything but funny. I can tell she's making a joke because she feels like she's supposed to. Knowing Mary Ann, she is holding the camera close to her, following her down the hallway, not ending the scene, hoping for more nervous chatter, even though I'm sure Lucy would like to yell, "Cut!"

In the next scene of the film, it is three months later. Lucy is back from her medical leave, working at CPEP again. She is wearing a scarf to cover her bald head, and her cheeks are hollowed.

Do You Want to Know a Secret?

It's the Bellevue holiday party, and Lucy has been back at the job for a short while. September and October were filled with neurosurgeries and radiation. Sadie gave birth to Billy in early November. He was named after Lucy's father, and his arrival was followed just two days later by her first round of chemotherapy. The tumors have been removed, and she is now on high-dose steroids and Dilantin to prevent seizures. The steroids are revving her up, making her hyper, almost hypomanic. She is way more irritable and impulsive than usual. At the party, Lucy nearly gets into a fistfight with one of the male nurses from the upstairs wards. He is antagonistic and inappropriate, which is typical for him, but then again, so is she. I try to run interference, keeping everyone calm, and the situation deflates eventually, but not before she invites him to step outside. It's a party; everyone's dressed up. Now is not the time to rumble, I plead.

I end up speaking to our boss, Dr. MacKenzie, later in the night. He is Lucy's supervisor, and I know they've spent a lot of time talking lately. In his late forties, with curly salt-and-pepper hair and glasses, he's so tall I have to crane my neck to establish eye contact. "I'm worried about Lucy. Have you noticed how reactive she is lately?" I ask.

"Well, you know Lucy," he responds, noncommittal. I don't know how much he knows about her situation. Does he know about the neurosurgery? The steroids? Does he know, but doesn't realize that I know? We are like two secret agents, wary of committing an act of treason.

"So you're not worried about her behavior?" I ask.

"Not any more than usual." He smiles.

"Okay, then." I leave it at that. I want to talk to someone who understands the situation, who knows what medicines she's taking. I want to tell him I'm worried the steroids are making her disinhibited and aggressive, but I don't. I have no idea what he knows and what he doesn't. I don't want to get her into trouble, but I'm afraid she's going to get herself into some.

I know that Lucy wants to keep her job, and I don't want to jeopardize that. She feels she has to keep working; she needs her medical benefits. Plus, she'd go crazy at home all day with nothing to do. She's already dissolved her private practice, referring many of her patients to me.

That was a big deal, Lucy closing down her practice. She was the one who helped me get mine up and running. Back when I was just starting out, she advised me on everything from my rates to malpractice insurance to office policy. The fact that I am now treating her patients sends us all a powerful message that she is ill. Her patients are in love with her; I am a facsimile only. They have this idea that when she gets well again, she'll reopen her practice and take them back into the fold.

I am playing along with this fantasy, because it's what feels right to all of us.

How to Save a Life

New Year's Eve 1998 is on a Thursday night, so I don't have to work. There are few things more depressing than watching the ball drop with downhearted and delusional patients: We crowd around the television, and when the lighted orb finally touches down in Times Square, there is the painfully awkward moment of deciding whom to kiss. The staff members hug one another, but the patients, all the lonely people, stand or sit, disconnected, forlorn.

The weekend after New Year's, there's not much action on Saturday night, but early in my shift on Sunday, we get two cases back-to-back: a man and a woman, related only by a random, horrific event.

A petite blonde in her twenties has been escorted here by MTA police and NYPD. She keeps repeating that she's missing a party with her family. I tell her she's lucky she's still alive to miss the party. The other pretty blond girl, the one standing next to her, waiting for the N train on the Twenty-third Street subway platform, won't be seeing her family again. My patient has just witnessed thirty-two-year-old Kendra Webdale being pushed into the path of an oncoming train.

Anyone waiting for a subway and seeing a man push a woman onto the tracks would be justifiably upset, but she has the added layer of survivor guilt to deal with. Why wasn't she chosen as a victim? Why does she get to go on with her life when Kendra cannot? She saw the man ask Kendra a question, get her attention in some way, and then push her with all his might. Did he ask for the time? Did he ask her if she was ready to die? In some way, my patient has been given a small gift, and I think over time she will come to appreciate this. She has been taught that anyone's life can be taken away in an instant—at least in this city it can—and she'd best make the most of her time here.

She calms down fairly quickly and leaves CPEP after a short interview and a call to her dad. The next patient to be seen is the subway conductor. He is unintentionally but effectively complicit in Kendra's murder, mowing her down with his oncoming train. The level of guilt he is dealing with is above and beyond my first patient's. There was absolutely nothing he could've done to stop the eighty thousand pounds of subway cars in the split-second before the impact, but it will likely take years for him to get the images out of his head. From his windowed control car, inches away, he has seen everything.

The resident working with me that night sees the conductor, and I sign off on both charts and T & R orders. When I talk to Vera, the head nurse for the night, about our two patients, I can't help but wonder out loud where the third is. What's taking so long for the cops to bring him in?

"So where's the pusher?" I say to the staff in the nurses' station.

"I don't know. Do you think he's one of ours?"

"He must be. I bet you anything he's a psych patient. Why aren't they bringing him in for clearance?"

I wait all night for the subway pusher to be brought in, but he never materializes on my shift. He shows up at Bellevue on Monday, when I'm not on shift. (I later find out that he did ask to be brought to the hospital, that he specifically asked to see a doctor while he was still on the subway platform. The cops held him for a day, to get his confession, I suppose.)

And he is one of ours. More than that, he's one of mine: Jonah Bergman. I remember him well. He was a sweetheart, meek and gentle when I interviewed him a few months before the attack. It's not that often I get a Jewish schizophrenic, and what's more, he had the exact same name as a childhood friend of mine. And this is how I am able to remember him immediately, his name, his face, his story. Because when he came in that first time, I took special care of him.

There's something about schizophrenia, how devastating it is, how relentless its course can be, that draws me to it. Those patients automatically win my sympathy. I spent extra time sitting with Jonah, making sure he felt safe inside the CPEP. I can tell you exactly where he sat, and I remember we talked about music. He was soft-spoken, he seemed very intelligent, and he smiled at me while we spoke. I admitted him to our EOU so we could observe him for a few days before we released him. That was well before the attack, so hopefully no one will be pointing the finger at Bellevue, because obviously, someone dropped the ball in terms of his psychiatric care.

At the time of the assault, he was just a few weeks out from an admission at North General. He was supposed to be transferred to a state hospital, but there were no beds available, so he was discharged to fend for himself at his apartment.

So what happened to him? Did he go off his meds? Or was he so sick that even though he was taking his medication, his symptoms broke through? I wonder how his family will take this terrible turn of events. I learned in the newspapers that Jonah started out so promising, going to Bronx Science, wanting to be a doctor like his father. He made the dean's list at Stonybrook his freshman year, but it all fell apart when he was a sophomore. That is often the case with schizophrenia. Everything is going along fine, and then it slowly disintegrates: the paranoia, the isolation, the voices. His illness has taken its toll on his family, I'm sure. It's devastating to have a child who is in and out of hospitals, too sick to finish college or work for a living. And now this. I know the Webdale family is suffering, but my heart goes out to the Bergmans as well.

Jonah is admitted to our forensic unit the day after the attack, and I go to visit him up there the next weekend. When I walk in, he is alone in a room on 19 West, sitting on his bed, staring at the doorway, motionless. He seems to remember me, and so I sit down to chat on his bed. He tells me what happened that Sunday, how he spent the day eating at McDonald's, hanging out at Virgin Records listening to music and watching the movies playing in the store. I ask him to tell me what happened on the N-R platform, and he says that he was overcome, possessed by a spirit that pushed the girl. He feels like it wasn't him, that some force came into his body and did this. He looks at me with a blank stare, barely blinking, his mouth slack.

"It wasn't really me that did it," he explains.

I let this go, since it is a complicated concept. Is he the same person when his symptoms are in check by the medication? How much responsibility does he have if he is "out of his mind" at the time of the attack?

"And what about now?" I ask him. "Do you know what will happen next?"

He seems to know he'll stay at Bellevue for a while, and then he'll be tried in court. If he's scared, he's not showing it to me. Actually, he shows very little emotion, which is the way it is for many people with schizophrenia. I can't tell for sure if some part of him knew what he was doing on that platform and he's making up the part about the spirit, or if he really was so psychotic that he shouldn't be blamed. Good thing it isn't my job to figure that out. I'm not sure anyone could know that with any certainty.

I head back down to CPEP to work my shift, saddened by it all.

Several months later, it's a Sunday night and I'm working again with my favorite social worker, Julia. She is a wonderfully kooky gal, always wearing bright lipstick and quirky outfits, often involving sequins and headbands, or at least a sequined headband. The nurses from 19 West call down to speak with her, since she is the only social worker in the hospital assigned to psychiatry. Jonah is going to court tomorrow and he just told the nurses he has nothing to wear.

Julia and I go to the clothes room on the ground floor. There is a bigger clothes room in the basement, but Julia doesn't have a key to that area. I have heard that it is an enormous space, filled with pants, shirts, coats, and shoes for the homeless patients who need clothing prior to discharge. I'm disappointed I won't be seeing it. The big clothes room has attained a mythic status over the years, and with Julia not having the proper key, it makes me start to question whether it actually exists at all. Luckily, Julia and I find what we're looking for in the smaller room. Among the several racks and shelves we find a tan sweater, a plaid button-down shirt, and a pair of pants that should hopefully fit Jonah. We take the outfit up to 19 West and he tries on the clothes. He looks fine, and Julia and I commend ourselves on our makeover, but I don't think it's going to help him. I am worried for him, but I can't tell if he's worried too, because of that impenetrable blank stare, the flat affect of schizophrenia that makes it so hard to discern what someone is feeling. That's going to hurt him when he testifies, I just know it.

His first trial for second degree murder results in a hung jury in November of 1999. His second trial in March of 2000 requires only one hour of jury deliberation to deliver a guilty verdict, sentencing him to twenty-five years to life. I am not involved in the trials, but I watch them from afar, in the press like everyone else. At his sentencing, his defense attorney summarizes, "He's not a monster, Judge. He's a shell of the man he used to be." The sentence is overturned later on a technicality involving a psychiatrist's testimony, and he needs to be tried a third time. It is only in October of 2006, nearly seven years later, that the case is finally settled. He pleads guilty and receives twenty-three years, plus five years of supervised time upon release.

The interesting thing that comes out of this whole ordeal, and which comes quite swiftly compared to Jonah's sentence, is legislation referred to as Kendra's Law, 9.60 of the New York State mental hygiene legal code, which provides for court-ordered outpatient treatment. Now, not only can a patient be committed to an inpatient hospital stay, he can be mandated to outpatient treatment and monitoring as well. The civil liberties ramifications are obvious, forcing someone to undergo psychiatric treatment for months on end whether they like it or not. There are people who think this legislation is unjust, but I believe the spirit of the law is right. Jonah fell through the cracks. Everyone seems to agree about this. He was mentally ill and needed more supervision, more continuity of care. He bounced from hospital to hospital, from clinic to clinic, and from one makeshift housing solution to the next.

What was missing was what Jonah needed most: someone who would take responsibility for him and take care of him. Like many people with chronic mental illness, he had a family that went by the wayside. For many reasons, parents and siblings get burnt out. It's exhausting to care for someone who can't care for himself, and mental illness lasts a lifetime. It's difficult for families to stand by and watch one of their own deteriorate, re-compensate, and deteriorate again, repeatedly. People with persistent mental illness that doesn't respond well to medication often leave their families and end up on the street, in shelters, or perhaps in group homes if they're lucky. The shelters are a mismatched combination of crowded and lonely. There's no solitude, no privacy, but there is also very little human connection to be found there. Most chronic patients end up warehoused in the shelters and the state hospitals, which are a lousy solution.

The bottom line is that there are fewer beds than there are patients, mostly due to President Kennedy's 1963 Community Mental Health Centers Act. This well-intentioned movement helped to spur deinstitutionalization. The decision was made, when effective antipsychotics became readily available, to close down the mammoth state hospitals that were only providing custodial care, not treatment, with the idea that their patients would be transitioned from the state hospitals to community-based care. Many of the state facilities were shuttered, but the community centers never fully materialized, mostly due to a "not in my backyard" mentality in the neighborhoods. Thus, the homeless mentally ill population was spawned. Over the years, many stopgap measures have been put into place, but often, the adult homes and other housing options are ineptly run, overburdened, and sparsely funded.

Jonah needed one treatment team to be responsible for him, to approximate a substitute family that would check up on him, make sure he was taking his medication and seeing his doctor. Kendra's Law will help to make sure this level of supervised outpatient treatment occurs, through a hearing and a court order. If a patient in the assisted outpatient treatment program fails to comply with the treatment plan, he can be brought into the hospital for an evaluation and potential admission.

If the state of Virginia had a version of Kendra's Law, then maybe the Virginia Tech shooter would have been receiving much-needed psychiatric treatment, instead of slowly simmering in his psychosis alone in his dorm room.

I appreciate that from a libertarian point of view, Kendra's Law is a little over-the-top, but from a psychiatric point of view, it's just what the doctor ordered, to help our patients who are getting substandard, poorly coordinated care. It is meant to keep them healthy, and to keep everyone else safe. Ultimately, it could prevent another young woman like Kendra Webdale from falling prey to the fallout of haphazard mental health care.

We can't put Pandora back in her box. The homeless mentally ill have been with us since the sixties. The sooner we provide for them, the more s the causes of their problems, the better for us all.

I Will

"Seventy-two and sunny, seventy-two and sunny." I repeat my mantra as I run my laps around the reservoir in Central Park. After months of nagging Jeremy, and then wisely backing off at his insistence, he finally popped the question on my birthday. I am getting married in the park in early May, in the Conservatory Garden, where they don't allow tents.

"What do people do if it rains?" I ask the woman in charge of booking the venue.

"They bring an umbrella," she answers in all seriousness.

I have embarked on an ambitious exercise program in order to look my best for the wedding. I was inspired by a patient at Bellevue who managed to get off drugs and alcohol. When I asked him how he did it, he told me his first step was to complete "ninety in ninety." He went to ninety AA meetings in ninety days. That got me thinking: *Do I have that kind of discipline? Is there anything I would do for ninety days in a row?* I decide to get in shape for the big day by doing ninety workouts in ninety days. For three months without fail I run, lift, swim laps, do a step class, go Rollerblading or biking. It has paid off: On the morning of my wedding, as I step on the scale, I have magically reached my goal weight. Equally miraculous is the forecast for the day: a high of seventy-two degrees, breezy, with ample sunshine. It's enough to make a gal thank her lucky stars. Add to that my bliss from finally passing my oral boards, and everything's coming up roses.

Jeremy and I have decided to make this wedding an intimate group effort. We've invited our friends and family to form the wedding band, take the pictures, bake the cake. I am excited about being serenaded by our closest friends, who will strum their guitars and sing Bob Dylan's "Make You Feel My Love," as we walk among the flowers to the makeshift altar, three steps underneath a metal archway covered with roses and vines. Our wedding party consists of our two eight-year-old nieces, Zaro and Violet (the "drymaids" in Violet's words), our two five-year-old nephews, Jake and Jonah (the "ring barriers"), and our three-year-old niece, Ivy, the flower girl.

The garden is at its peak of perfection. The cherry blossoms are floating down like snowflakes in the wind. Hundreds of tulips in purple and pink line the plaza where the ceremony will take place. Ivy has been carrying a single purple tulip tightly in her fist, waiting for her big moment when she will start the procession. I stand behind the shrubs, hiding from the guests, and taking the occasional peek at them while talking mindlessly with my parents, who will escort me down the aisle.

Lucy has come with Sadie. Other people from Bellevue can come to the reception, but only Lucy is invited to the ceremony. She has warned me that she will be wearing her festive wig today. She owns two wigs, one worse than the other, and on this day, it appears to me she has worn the larger of the two. It is auburn; the long tresses ending in big curls. It is God-awful, and I love her for it, for not caring, for wearing it anyway, for slapping on some makeup and lipstick and dragging her sorry ass to the garden to share this day with me.

After a meltdown about losing her tulip, Ivy walks hand in hand with her mother down the aisle, and so the wedding begins.

It's a glorious day, the breeze blowing my veil around, and also blowing the words of the rabbi away. The guests wait patiently as the sermon drags on, and eventually, Jeremy stomps on the glass, counts the band off for the recessional ("The Lucky One," by Freedy Johnston), and kisses me. The crowd cheers and claps as we kiss, and hug, and kiss some more.

I am insanely happy.

All Together Now

Lucy has invited all the CPEP faculty out to her house in the Hamptons for dinner and to see the fireworks for the Fourth of July. It's the medical new year, and there are fresh faculty members to get to know. Some of the doctors are staying over at Lucy and Sadie's house along with me and Jeremy, while others are sleeping at nearby hotels. It is the first time that we are all doing something social, as if we were a family, and the gathering has a warm and festive air to it.

When Jeremy and I arrive, Lucy is trying to corral her son Billy into a highchair so she can give him his lunch. I am mesmerized as I watch my pal with her boy, wearing an "I Love My Two Mommies" T-shirt. I can't look at Billy's T-shirt without thinking of Lucy's cancer, and wondering how soon he'll be down to one mommy.

We are outside in the sunshine as we gape at Billy, who is a beautiful babbling boy. He crawls, he smiles, he is the star of the day, eclipsing all others around him. Lucy feeds Billy with a spoon, making hysterical faces to get him to open his mouth. She is wearing a plaid hat over her bald head instead of her usual scarf or wig. She seems more relaxed and happier than I've ever seen her.

A new attending, Michelle, is just meeting us all. She is fresh out of a residency in Massachusetts, and seems very young; she's wearing thick pancake makeup, and I wonder what she's trying to cover up. I sneak a peek at her bedroom, downstairs from Lucy and Sadie's. There is a stuffed animal on the pillow. *Is this gal for real? She brought her teddy to the sleepover?*

Throughout the holiday weekend, we rotate in front of the television; JFK Jr.'s plane has gone down on its way to Martha's Vineyard. I imagine most of America glued to their televisions instead of outside at their barbecues as the network tantalizingly teases and threatens to broadcast the recovery of the bodies.

On Saturday night (I have asked someone to take my shift at CPEP), we eat outside in the backyard under the stars. Sadie has marinated huge porterhouse steaks in a balsamic vinaigrette.

"You guys, there aren't enough steaks for everyone to have their own," says Lucy. "Some of you have to share."

"Daniel and I can share!" I volunteer. I turn to him. "Do you like it medium rare?"

Daniel is not happy about this, but doesn't come right out and say it. I've announced this, to the table full of physicians, to assert that we are friends, that we have a history together. I want Lucy to know that I am down with her right-hand man. Lucy, though bald and thin, still has a tremendous vitality and presence, but it's becoming clear to most of us that Daniel will eventually succeed her and become the new director. He is being "groomed" and trained by Lucy as she prepares for her departure. He has already filled in for her whenever she is out sick, which is becoming more frequent. I'm trying to get used to the idea that he will eventually become my boss.

By answering Lucy's call and volunteering to share with Daniel, I'm trying to let the other doctors know that I'm in the upper echelon of the power structure at CPEP, that Lucy and Daniel, the director and assistant director, are my friends and colleagues, not my superiors. Here's another thought: I am attempting to bond with Daniel on a masculine level. The steak, a symbol of manhood: We are sharing the kill, predators flush with the thrill of the hunt, putting down our weapons for the feast. Or maybe it has something to do with laying claim to Lucy? Maybe she is the prize, and I am offering to divide it. We are marking our territory over her, snarling animals fighting for our share of the prey, carving her up between us like divided turf.

Whatever it may mean (sometimes being a shrink means you think too much about this stuff) Daniel wants his own steak, of course. What man wouldn't? And we are not a couple. We are not even good friends, really. Why do I offer to share with him instead of with Jeremy? My brand-new husband is sitting a few seats down from Lucy, who is at the head of the table. I am sitting next to Daniel at the foot of the table. Daniel, trying to analyze my chumminess, I imagine, is not particularly interested in joining my newly created pecking order, but we share the steak nonetheless.

After dinner we all walk down to the edge of the bay. Sadie and Lucy's neighbors have graciously offered us the use of their lawn and chairs, and we have a fabulous view.

And then come the fireworks.

Tell Me Why

I spend a slew of Mondays with Mary, my dutiful shrink, who, along with me, is getting used to the idea that Lucy will lose her drawn-out war, her body occupied by an unwanted enemy.

I cannot get past how guilty I feel. I'm fine but my friend is sick. And it's more complicated than that, because I am now four months pregnant. Lucy is dying and I am blooming with life. It is an ironic and painfully awkward juxtaposition. She is wasting away and losing hope, as I enlarge with the promise of the future looking the very picture of health. It makes me feel greedy, as if I'm taking more than my share from the dinner platter, and there really isn't enough to go around.

Mary points out that this is survivor guilt, plain and simple. She helps me to understand it more fully, how it resonates with my issues from childhood, beating out my sisters to get more than my share from our father. I have a similar discomfort being healthy and wealthy among the sick, poor, and homeless Bellevue patients. I won't wear my diamond engagement ring to work, and I still feel guilty that I have my freedom while they stay locked up in the hospital.

I hate feeling overstuffed among the hungry. I prefer things to be evenly divided. Gluttonous, I'm relishing eating for two, while Lucy can barely chew her cheese omelet because it hurts her head. We are at the Bellevue coffee shop one Monday morning after sign-out, old friends catching up on this and that. As usual, I cannot bring myself to discuss any of the really important matters with Lucy, but finally she breaks the ice.

"Julie, you know, you and I are at radically different points in our lives," she says to me. The imbalance has been impossible to ignore, of course, and I am grateful that she is bringing it up at last, tossing it across the table to me like a beach ball, breezily.

"I've noticed it too, dude," I answer back. "It is nothing if not completely fucked up." We stare meaningfully at each other for a long moment, and then at last begin to have a real conversation, slowly working our way toward the meat of the matter. We both have a tendency to play up our macho butch angle with each other. It always worked on others, getting their attention and admiration, and we use it on each other to reinforce our bond. But now it feels like it's time to get more girly. More real.

Instead of talking about her cancer and failing health, how brave she is in the face of death, we begin to talk of children and motherhood. I tell her how I stare at the little girls in pink in their ballet class before I go into my Pilates class, wanting a little girl of my own, but afraid of how hard it will be: The mother-daughter dramas are inevitable, and if there's anything to karma, my payback will be a bitch, just as I was to my mother in my teens. She tells me that Mary has a daughter, and I admit to Lucy that Mary and I have been spending countless hours talking about the what-ifs of raising a girl, but I do not tell her we spend the rest of the time discussing her cancer and my guilt.

I tell her she's lucky she has a son, that they are easier to handle, at least emotionally, and Lucy confides in me that lately she has been afraid to bond with Billy. She is pulling back from everyone now, resigning herself to her prognosis. It's only a matter of time, in her eyes, before she checks out, so she's starting to pack up early. She knows she's doing it, and defends her behavior to me. Part of it is protecting herself, and part of it, she feels, is protecting Billy from loving her too much so it won't hurt him quite as much when she abandons him.

She's wrong, of course. I want to tell her not to shortchange herself, or him, and that she should maximize whatever time she has left, to love and be loved. That's all that life can really give us: time, joy, love. Being fully present is the best gift she can give him. But I don't want to turn into that naive little Kansan Pollyanna with her again; I want to stay strong for her, to mirror her bravery, and so I mostly remain silent. The thing that binds us, the persona we share, is our macho exterior. If I shed it, I fear, we will have no special connection anymore, and even less common ground on which to rest.

Having My Baby

Monday, May 15, 2000. I leave Bellevue to head to the Upper West Side for an appointment with my midwife; I am thirty-seven weeks pregnant, but the baby's head has already dropped into position. I never thought I'd complain so much about having a head between my legs.

Later that same day, while reading a *New Yorker* in Mary's waiting room, I have some cramps and my underwear becomes wet. I get very excited, believing this to signify the onset of labor. I leave Mary's office before our hour is up, too excited to sit still. Jeremy is in Indianapolis on business, taking pictures of various tourist destinations in the city for an ad campaign. I call his hotel to let him know what's going on. "I'll check the flight schedule," he promises.

For the rest of the day I feel only cramping that is irregular and mild. Still, I stop by the birthing center for a quick exam. The midwife on duty confirms that I have lost my mucous plug and warns me that there may not be much time between my water breaking and the delivery because the head is so low. She agrees that I'm in early labor but can't say how soon I will deliver.

"My husband is away on business," I say. "He's shooting a baby elephant at a zoo tomorrow."

"Shooting?" she asks.

"Photographing," I explain.

The rhythm of our speech resonates with something in my psyche.

Then, like a bomb exploding in my face, I have a flashback of the assault that happened years ago. *"Feigning?" he asks. "Faking," I explain.* And then the fist.

I call Jeremy during the cab ride home and give him an update. He decides to fly back early the next morning, skipping the baby elephant. Once home, I follow the midwife's advice for stalling labor and pour myself a couple of fingers of Bushmills. Lying in bed, I worry about all the things that can go wrong with my baby. Most pregnant woman fear birth defects; I fear schizophrenia. I know how fragile the brain is. My child will be fine until turning eighteen or so, and then everything will slowly unravel, and I'll be powerless to stop it.

The next day, Tuesday, I cancel all my plans for the week, including my private practice patients on Friday. I put my friend Kate, a veteran of two home births, on standby in case Jeremy doesn't make it home in time. I am all set to deliver. Only nothing really happens after that. Jeremy lands around noon and things have quieted down with my pelvis.

"Those contractions sound like classic Braxton-Hicks to me," Joan tells me when I call her to check in. "You're not in labor at all. It still could be weeks until you deliver."

This is unacceptable to me. I ask her about ways to help speed labor along. "Listen, Julie, I'm not going to advise you on how to induce labor. You're only thirty-eight weeks. The longer you can gestate, the better for the baby."

I know she's right, but I am discouraged. I talk to Kate who tells me that childbirth is like a ride; I can't drive it. I have to let go and allow my body to be in charge.

A week goes by. I speak to everyone I have ever known on the phone. I cook and freeze enough food to last us a month. I work incessantly on a book I'm editing about the drug Ecstasy, and have long meetings on the phone with the editor in Vermont. Tonight there's a party at Grand Central Station celebrating the 150th anniversary of *Harper's Magazine*. We know it is our last chance to go out as a childless couple, and we are glad, for once, that the baby hasn't yet arrived.

At the party is Spalding Gray, an actor who performs wonderful monologues off-Broadway and in films. I am a fan who has become a friend. When I met him at an earlier *Harper's* party, I was too shy to speak to him for very long, but I did manage to ask him to blurb my Ecstasy book, and he graciously agreed. After that, I ended up spending most of my time talking to his wife, Kathie, who was vivacious and garrulous. Over the years, we have become friends. She is with him on the dance floor now, and we go out to join them. Spalding is pretty spazzy and entertaining when he dances, and I laugh a lot while trying to keep up. I feel as if I am shaking the baby down, helping it to drop into place with every shimmy.

The next morning I have another appointment with the midwife. I go home and have some mild cramping which intensifies later in the day. When my water breaks, I immediately call Joan, who says, "Okay, call me back when your contractions are four minutes apart. Wait until the contractions last a full minute and are so intense you can't do anything during one. Make sure you're hydrated. Check back in with me around six o'clock."

It is two-thirty in the afternoon. I call Jeremy and my mother, then I figure I'd better grab a shower before we go to the birthing center. During the shower I have four contractions. As I towel off, I have yet another contraction.

How long was my shower if I've had five contractions? Even if it was a twenty-minute shower, they're four minutes apart, and I wasn't in there that long. I start to take notes, recording the time and length of each contraction. By three-fifteen, I realize they are coming every ninety seconds or so, and consistently last thirty-five to forty seconds. They are picking up in intensity, so I decide to call Joan again.

Since she just heard from me less than an hour ago, Joan thinks it's still early in my labor. She is very focused on the fact that my contractions are not lasting a full minute. "Lie down and do your hypno-birthing exercises and relax for a little while."

"Joan, I need to be where you are. I'll relax once I'm at the birthing center. These contractions are coming fast, and they're intense, and I would feel much more comfortable if I could labor at the hospital instead of at my apartment. I'd feel better getting into a trance there instead of here."

She is still resistant, challenging me. "Isn't the whole point of doing hypnosis that you can relax anywhere?" But I am not to be dissuaded. Reluctantly she tells me, "Look, if you really want to come in, you can, because there's nothing much happening here at the center. If you're only two centimeters, I'll send you down the street to see a movie."

"If I'm only two centimeters when I get there, you can send me home," I tell her.

When I get off the phone, I stand staring for a moment, replaying the conversation in my mind. She is acting like me, the way I do at the hospital. She's being tough and defiant, downplaying my experience, and I am cast in a different role, the one where I have to defend my symptoms, and I have no power. I still have to convince Jeremy, who's home by now but wants to believe the midwife—the professional. She knows her job, and if she's telling me it's too early to come in, then maybe it is.

"We need to go *now!*" I tell him.

We finish packing our bags and head down to the street to find a cab. It is three-thirty in the afternoon, the Thursday before Memorial Day, and the traffic is heavy on Ninety-sixth Street. I lean against a parking meter and then a fire hydrant during my contractions. When they hit, I am doubled over in pain. They have a crescendo to them, and a long plateau. Then, just as I feel I can't take it another second, they subside, and I can straighten up and walk.

Two Caribbean women walk by, pointing me out in their lilting island accents, "She look like she ready to drop." They see me hunched over and ask if I need any help, telling me I should take an ambulance, not a cab, to the hospital.

"I'm fine between the contractions," I say to them, and they smile and nod vigorously with understanding. I am about to join their club. Millions of women have done what I am now doing. I'm being hazed into a sorority, the League of Women Birthers.

The cab ride to the hospital takes around fifteen minutes, and I have at least five contractions as we careen down Fifth Avenue. Each one is getting more intense, coming on the heels of the previous one, and I am getting more irritable.

At the entrance to the hospital, I have to stop in the middle of the lobby before the security guard's station, because I am having another huge contraction and am paralyzed. A young nurse shows us to a birthing room. I walk in and start to take off my shoes, my watch, my clothes. I need to be naked, and I can't stand still. I alternate between shifting my weight from leg to leg and shaking out each leg in succession. I am the size of a manatee, but I can still do a great shimmy.

"Relax," the nurse tells me. "You're too tense," she says while massaging my shoulders and neck. *I'm a teepee, I'm a wigwam,* I think to myself, the oldest joke I know. My shoulders are bunched up toward my ears, it's true, but I am experiencing a vice gripping my pelvis, and I've had no success unwinding so far. All the hypno-birthing preparation and the reading about relaxing through the contractions has been wasted on me. It's just not possible.

Joan comes in to examine me, and she is wearing scrubs. "Okay, let's stop playing around now," she says. I have no idea what she's talking about. "You're eight centimeters."

Those three lovely words. "So you wanna send me to a movie now?" I ask her, a tad angry, but trying to keep it light. She is in the scrubs, and I am naked. Clearly I need to subordinate myself to her and to the process at hand.

And right there, in the birthing center of Saint Luke's Hospital, I have a medium-sized epiphany that has nothing to do with labor and delivery. She didn't believe me when I called her. My clinician has failed me, and it hurt. Finally I realize, like never before, that I absolutely need to listen to my patients better, to be more open to believing their side of the story, trust that they need my care, and not always assume that I know more than they do. Just because I'm in a position of power does not mean I have to wield it, creating an impenetrable fortress.

Needless to say, I can't dwell on this revelation. I am already feeling an urge to push, and I ask her if it's okay.

"Do what your body tells you," she coos.

With the contractions, I sneak in a squeeze here and there, a way to push against the pain.

"Let the baby come down," she whispers.

I move around on the bed, but I can't get comfortable. No position brings any kind of relief. The nurse wipes a cold compress on my head every once in a while and I keep thanking her, because it feels so good.

I have only put in a few pushes, sometimes waiting out a contraction or two before I push again, and already Joan is telling Jeremy to look so he can see the head.

"Camera," I wheeze, and my photographer husband obliges.

It takes me a while to get better at pushing. It is exhausting, and it hurts, and I have a strong instinct to avoid doing something that both requires energy and brings me enormous pain.

"Charley horse!" I groan, as my left thigh seizes up, hard and tight. It distracts me entirely from my all-consuming task, forcing another person out of my body. The nurse massages my thigh expertly as the pain subsides.

"I don't want to tear," I remind Joan.

"Just don't push if you feel a burning," she replies.

After a few more pushes, it burns, and I tell her so.

"Wait. Breathe. Don't push."

I wait. I pant, just like they do in the movies. Pretty soon I can't not push. I have to push, the way I would have to breathe if I held my breath. There is a white hot ring of fire between my legs and I need to extinguish it. Joan tells me to go ahead and push, even though it is burning. And then I feel myself tear. It is unmistakable—a separate, serrated layer of fire-engine red pain on top of the white-hot searing pain.

"I'm tearing, aren't I?" I ask her, unable to conceal the panic in my voice.

"Yes," she answers matter-of-factly. She tells me where, and I ask her a few questions, slipping into doctor mode for just a minute, to make sure all the important parts are still intact. She assures me they are.

"What do I do?" I ask her.

"Push!" she answers.

The head is out. I can see it between my legs as Joan tells me to stop pushing for a minute. I pant again, glad for the respite as she suctions the baby's mouth. But I know from my obstetrics rotations in medical school that the shoulders are the killers, the widest part of the baby. I start pushing again and, sure enough, the pain becomes even more intense. "Joan, I don't care what you have to do, just get this thing out of me!" I am yelling, panicking, on the edge of something, tipping, falling.

And then the baby is out, slippery, bluish, covered in mucus, blood, and creamy white vernix.

"It's a girl!" Joan announces.

I had forgotten that we didn't know the sex of the baby, or even that we get to find out; it had been obscured by the pain. A girl. It's what we both wanted. I break into a wide grin as I meet Jeremy's eyes.

Onto my chest is placed my baby girl, all purple and cheesy and slimy and warm, with her eyes wide open.

Jeremy cuts the cord once it stops pulsating. After Joan is done sewing, I can finally sit up and relax with my baby girl.

Later, as I unpack my overnight bag, Jeremy and I have a good laugh at all I had stowed in the bag to occupy our time during the labor: scented candles, massage oil, relaxation tapes. Molly, my lovely, perfect, beautiful new daughter, took all of forty-five minutes to come into the world from the moment we walked into the hospital.

You're Gonna Make Me Lonesome
When You Go

I take three months off for maternity leave, and we spend part of the summer on Cape Cod. When I return to the city, I stop by Daniel's apartment, one block from my own, to show off my new baby. When she starts fussing and I begin to nurse her, I am surprised by Daniel's blush as he turns away. Any dirty jokes we may have shared over the years as I pretended to be one of the guys are now completely off-limits. I have become a mother in his eyes, and if there's one thing I know about Daniel, he reveres his mother.

I start back up at work in September, delighted to see how Lucy's cancer has responded to a new medication called Herceptin. It puts her into a remission of sorts, and so she continues to come to work nearly every day. I get the feeling that she is pulling back from our friendship, though, and I take her cue. As the months go by, I work my weekends, see her briefly on Monday mornings, and pull back as well. With a new baby at home, it's easy to lose touch. Too easy. And too convenient an excuse not to do something that is painful for me.

Mary and I move into a holding pattern of our own. My life is more settled now. Jeremy and I have eased into our roles as parents, and I am no longer taunting the patients and putting my safety in jeopardy. We've mined my childhood and CPEP behavior for three years, and the sessions are starting to seem like a coda to a song, repeating and fading.

Termination is a big deal with therapists; typically, there are months spent discussing how the patient feels about stopping the sessions. Abandonment issues always crop up in these situations. I am actually more worried about how Mary will take my leaving, and much less worried about how I will do without her. I attempt to terminate much more quickly than usual, trying to wrap things up in one session.

"I was watching this movie, and there was a little girl trying to learn how to ride a bicycle. The father teaching her was running alongside her, helping to steady her, and once the girl had enough speed and balance on the bike, he let go. As the girl wobbled away, I started to get a little teary." I stop for effect here. "I realized I was like that girl, and you were the grown-up helping me learn how to ride my bike. Well, now I think I can do it on my own. I think I can take it from here."

Mary looks at me skeptically. At least I think it's skeptically. "What are you getting at, Julie?"

"I think I'm ready to end our therapy," I state, with as much assuredness as I can muster. If she detects any hesitance, she'll pounce on it, and we'll have to discuss this ad infinitum.

"I think you may be ready too," she replies.

Wow. Does this mean I'm fixed?

We spend two more Mondays wrapping up, summarizing and solidifying all I have learned in her office. Mary assures me I can always come back to her if I need to in the future, and I thank her profusely for all she has done for me.

When Lucy develops pneumonia during the winter and ends up in the hospital again, I don't go to visit her. I assume it is a small fire to be put out, and then she'll be back to business as usual. I don't realize that she is seriously ill, or else I'm merely pretending that it isn't a dire situation just yet. I tell myself that I need to get home to my daughter Molly after my long nights away. I need to nurse her and feel her in my arms again. On my drive home from Bellevue, I go right by the NYU hospital where Lucy is, but I don't take the time to stop in and sit with her.

I convince myself and all the other CPEP staff that this isn't the final round, that they haven't seen the last of Lucy Jones. At a faculty meeting, when the issue of Lucy's health arises, I assure everyone that she's not dying anytime soon, that she'll probably be back at work in a few weeks.

Daniel, who is now running the show in her absence, glares at me, to let me know this is an unreasonable thing to say, that I shouldn't assure them of her resilience at this stage of the game. He's been going to visit her most days after work, to keep her briefed on what's happening at Bellevue, and also just to be with her, which is what I should have been doing. He is much more up-to-date on her current medical situation.

So is it getting close to the end? My mind starts racing. What does Daniel's glare mean? That if I had been sitting at her bedside, I'd have understood her medical condition as accurately as he does? I honestly thought she wasn't that sick yet. Was that just wishful thinking, or more precisely, denial? Does he think she's going to die soon? I take his glare to mean: You should know this as well as I do. You are failing her as a friend.

And still I avoid going to visit her.

I am insulating myself, I know, but it hurts too much to see her so sick. Her star is fading, receding, and I cannot bear it. I can't fix it. I can't control it. I turn away to protect myself, even though I know it is selfish. When Sadie confronts me with my absence, I have no excuse for my behavior. I don't fully understand why I'm at such a loss for how I should be acting. It's as if I've used up all my emotional intelligence at the office and have none left over when I get home. Everyday life is just as complex as what I deal with at CPEP, but I am ill-equipped when out of my element.

Sadie is with her day and night, a steadfast companion. She leaves Billy with a sitter and sleeps next to Lucy. What can I do to prove my allegiance except to be there for her too?

I've already talked to Mary about it incessantly; at this point, there's only one thing left to do: go.

I finally make my way to the NYU hospital. I'd visited her there when she had her secret brain surgery, but that had been nearly a year ago. I'd brought her a plant then, a small chili pepper bush, with multiple red and orange peppers coming off the greenery at various angles. I thought it was a good symbol of her feistiness. Now, when I go to visit her in the ICU, I am empty-handed. I bring nothing to the table.

The unsinkable Lucy Jones is on a respirator. She is awake, but she cannot speak. I feel awkward and terrible as I rack my brain for things to fill my side of the one-sided conversation. I tell her about some inane gossip at work. I show her a flyer honoring Valerie, one of our favorite social workers, as employee of the month. None of this means a damn thing. She is fighting for her life and I have nothing to offer, not even a worthwhile distraction.

There is a book on the windowsill, and I flip through it as I take a break from my monologues. The book cover says *Worst Case Scenario Survival Handbook.* I leaf through it, and there is advice for all sorts of difficult situations: what to do if you are attacked by a bear, or if you are lost in the desert. Of course, there is no advice for how to act when your friend is dying. I become engrossed in the book when I am interrupted by a chirpy voice.

"Hi, Lucy! How's Billy?" asks the nurse, as she checks the monitors and documents the patient's blood pressure, her respirator settings. Lucy smiles and nods. Every nurse asks Lucy the same thing. There are pictures of her son up on the walls, and everyone knows his name is Billy. So they pretend they're friends with her and they know her son. It is maddening, but I don't know whether it's bothering Lucy. I want to ask her, but it seems too complicated for her to answer. She can write a word or two on the small chalkboard by her bed, she can nod yes or no, but we can't get into the intricacies of the nurses' behaviors, the little tricks of connection they use that nonetheless add up to genuine acts of kindness and compassion. I don't even know if she's picked up on it. I'm just not sure how with it she still is, if her searing intellect is still on fire.

After one more stab at failed small talk, I leave the ICU, telling her I'll be back, but I don't say when. I don't know if I'll feel capable of seeing her deteriorate even further. I want to have the healthy, strong, bullish Lucy in my head to keep me company when she's gone, not this one.

A week later, I visit Lucy one more time in the ICU. She has just been wheeled back into the room from having a CT scan of her torso. She is sedated in the bed. Her feet look flaccid, her lax toes pointed toward the wall instead of flexed toward the ceiling, and it strikes me as a bad sign. Since Lucy is sleeping, I go find Sadie in the lounge. We sit together and talk for a bit, and then Lucy's doctor comes over to speak with us. He's just seen her CT scan. He makes it clear that there's not much else he can do. The cancer has taken over Lucy's liver. I sit quietly next to Sadie for a moment and then say, "I'm just going to go say good-bye to her."

"You think she's going to die?" Sadie asks, panicked.

"I'm just going to say good-bye for now," I explain as I head back to her room. She is still asleep, or perhaps unconscious, as I kiss her cool forehead. It is the last time I see her.

Sadie calls me a few days later and wants my help. She wants Lucy to get an emergency liver transplant. She has Daniel calling the transplant service at Mount Sinai to see if this is possible. She also wants to get Lucy back on chemotherapy and is enlisting Daniel and me to call several drug companies to release experimental medicines for breast cancer.

These are all "Hail Mary passes" as far as I am concerned, and I have resigned myself to the fact that Lucy will die any day now, but Sadie is not ready to let go. Lucy was very clear with Sadie that she wanted everything done. She is not a "do not resuscitate." She is a "fight tooth and nail to pull out of a nosedive." I indulge Sadie's request, because at least now there's something I can do. I sit on my couch and call Astra-Zeneca, Novartis, and Bristol-Meyers-Squibb, talking to oncology researchers willing to part with some experimental potion. I get one man on the phone who is very kind and concerned, and he faxes me some forms for Lucy's oncologist to fill out to get a "compassionate use protocol" up and running. By the time he calls back asking for follow up, it is too late, as I knew it would be.

Now You're Gone

Sadie calls me the day that Lucy dies, Saturday, March 24, 2001. I am upstate at the house, which Jeremy and I bought in 1999. She tells me what it was like at the very end, though I can't bear to hear it. I pull the phone away from my ear as she conveys the details of her death.

I drive down to the city and head into work a few hours later. I leave a couple of messages with Daniel saying I need to speak with him, but he doesn't return my calls. Saturday night, and again on Sunday night, I spend most of my shifts breaking the news to the nurses, psych techs, social workers, clerks—anyone who knows and loves Lucy, which is everyone.

On Monday morning just before rounds start, Daniel comes in and makes the official announcement. There will be a private funeral service, and then later a more public memorial. Daniel says he isn't sure if the family wants flowers or donations, and I make the mistake of interrupting him to say that I have the name and number of a florist near Lucy's house in East Hampton.

"Can I finish, please?" he asks angrily, and my eyes tear up. He is furious with me for interrupting him, and my shame liquefies and pools on the edges of my lower lids.

I am so raw with her loss. All weekend, every time I passed by her office door on the way to my office, the waterworks would come right on cue. It doesn't take much now, in front of everyone at rounds, for me to start up all over again.

I am upset that my friend is gone, bitter that her life was cut short, and for a moment, like an angry child, I wish it were Daniel instead. When he is done with his speech and it is my turn to give the morning report, I can't speak. Dave, Daniel's right-hand man, is sitting next to me and I can't tell if he feels sorry for me, or thinks I am a stupid bitch for interrupting Daniel. All I know is he can see my tears. I stare down at my blurry paper willing them away so I can give sign-out.

I drive out to Long Island for the funeral with Jeremy and Molly, not yet one year old, and we stop at the ocean before going to the church. The sand is littered with starfish, more than I have ever seen. It is a blustery spring day, and the waves are high in the wind. I pick up four starfish, two big ones and two little ones. Years later, when I am trying to conceive my second child, I will stand in front of the four starfish on my windowsill and concentrate on a fourth member of my family, offering up a prayer to Lucy, telling her that I still miss her, and chanting to myself, "Mommy, daddy, daughter, son."

We arrive a bit late, thanks to screwy directions from Mapquest. We sit in the back, apart from my colleagues, who are all sitting together. As the funeral progresses, I cannot shake the feeling that I have been os-tracized by my fellow physicians and their mates. We have traveled here separately, we are sitting separately, and I have the bitter feeling that I don't belong in their little clique. It is a way to distract myself from the business at hand, mourning.

At the back of the small church, Molly is playing with Billy. Lucy would have been pleased to see them on the carpeted floor next to each other. Why didn't we ever get our kids together? Was she too sick by the time Molly was born, or did I become too busy being a working mother? I feel awful that we never tried to orchestrate it. I cheated my-self out of having more good times with her, and now I have no more chances to make things right.

During his eulogy, the minister does a good job of acknowledging the emotions of guilt and anger that always surround a death that comes too early in life. I am angry that she has been taken away, and Lucy was angry that she had to leave, and I am glad that anger is a recurring theme as peo-ple get up to speak. (When I speak at the public memorial months later, the anger that is still so vivid in my mind will be a major theme of my eu-logy.) We are also being regaled with some funny anecdotes from the dais, and people are laughing, which I'm sure Lucy would have wanted.

There is a long drive from the church to a protected cove that Lucy thought was especially beautiful, where Sadie wants to say a few words. I remember Lucy talking about kayaking in that cove this past summer, and how she was afraid it would be her last. She said it made her appreciate the sunsets more.

The limo drivers get lost on the way to the beach; the whole line of cars in the funeral procession has to make a U-turn, and it adds another layer of levity to the day's events. Later in the day nearly everyone notes how Lucy would have gotten a kick out of our getting lost en masse.

"Care to join us down here, Julie?" Sadie asks as I lag behind the crowd at the shore. Still feeling ostracized, I am defending myself from feeling left out by a preemptive aloofness. I apologize as I close in on the huddle standing on the wet sand.

We all have white flowers in our hands. We are supposed to throw them onto the water to symbolize our letting go, or saying good-bye, or something. It is windy and absurdly difficult to toss the flowers into the water. When they finally land in the ocean, the tide carries the flowers back to us, not out to sea. I know Lucy would've loved that too, rejecting our mourning, mocking our symbolic flower-tossing. You can't conquer the wind and the tides; nature triumphs over our puny plans. Death trumps all.

After the gathering at the bay, we go back to Lucy and Sadie's house. Sadie is doing a private burial so we don't go to the cemetery, which is fine with me. The part where the casket is lowered into the ground would have delivered a bone-crushing sense of loss and finality.

"How're you doing, buddy?" Daniel asks me as he puts his arm around me in the backyard.

"Pretty good, considering my pally just died," I choke out.

"I know. But it wasn't her. At the end. It wasn't her," Daniel says.

I have no response to what he's saying beyond a grunt of acknowledgment. Daniel is trying to comfort me, I suppose, the way he comforts himself, with a shot of denial, but I don't know where to start in continuing this conversation.

This is the closest we'll be, arm in arm. Things will disintegrate between us from here on out.

Let Him Eat Steak

Daniel has settled into the work of being the new CPEP director. It's a lousy position to be in, with the typical managerial dilemma: There's no pleasing everybody. He needs to meet the demands of the administration, first and foremost, but the CPEP staff assume his sole mission is to make them happy. He's being pulled in different directions by nearly everyone, and I'm just trying to stay out of his way.

This turns out to be impossible, because he wants more than that from me. As far as I can tell, in his new position as my superior, he wants me to kiss his ass. He pulls me into his office after a Monday morning sign-out, to yell at me for some perceived slight. I did not defer to him enough when he added his two cents on one of my case presentations, or I questioned the relevance of his interruption, as opposed to commending him for his incisive commentary. It's never going to be enough for him, I'm afraid. He needs a certain amount of public display of admiration to fuel his ego, and I can't pretend I have the regard for him that I did for Lucy.

"When we are in morning rounds, I expect you to treat me with respect," he warns, sounding an awful lot like my mom used to when I was thirteen. "Like it or not, I am the director now. And if I bring up a teaching point in rounds, you get behind it, don't roll your eyes or plow ahead to the next case."

"And?"

"And, you don't *tell* me when you're taking time off, you *ask* me to sign your vacation paperwork."

When Lucy was in charge, we were chums. I handed her my form and she signed it. She wouldn't have bothered to differentiate between telling and asking, and neither would I. And I did not need to subordinate myself to her. She didn't require it, first of all, and second, I had the utmost respect for her. I was in awe of her, basically. My feelings for Daniel border on disdain. Feigning adulation isn't going to be easy, and it seems like a nonnegotiable requirement for him.

"I'm your boss now, Julie. If you don't like it, you don't have to stay here." So there it is. *This town ain't big enough for the both of us. Danny boy, this is a showdown.*

"Why don't *you* leave?" I challenge, raising my voice. "I like my job. I'm happy here. And the people I work with happen to like me. You, they're not so crazy about."

He stares at me for a long time and says nothing. "I have no plans to leave this position anytime soon," he tells me, glaring.

"Great," I say. "Fine." I stall. I've got nothing. "Well, if we're both going to stay, we're obviously going to have to find a way to get along. I can try to be more subordinate in front of other people, if it'll help," I offer. I want him to know I'm on to him, how he likes to feel like the boss, how he seems to get off on the hierarchy. That I need to let the other worker bees know that I am another drone like them, and he is the queen. Otherwise, these private battles and public displays of dominance will likely continue.

"That's a good place to start," he accepts. Then he offers me a bone. "There's something else you should know. I totally covered your ass last week, so it's not like I don't look out for my own."

"What are you talking about?" *He's got my back? Is this possible?*

"That woman you kicked out of the nondetainable area last weekend?"

"Yeah . . ." I answer hesitantly. *Who did I kick out last weekend? That hysterical lady?*

"She was found in the lobby and brought to AES a little while afterwards. Tylenol overdose."

"Oh, Jesus. She was a walk-in, and she was crying like mad, saying she didn't want to be seen, she'd changed her mind. So I told her she could go. She walks in, she can walk out."

"Not necessarily. This is why you're never supposed to turn people away. You'll miss things if you don't interview them. You know that." He stares at me accusingly, and I know he is completely right. I can't possibly rationalize what I did and we both know it. Anyone that distraught should have been ushered through the doors and fully evaluated, but I couldn't deal with her level of drama, with the noise of it, and when she said she wanted to turn around and walk out the door, I was relieved.

I have screwed up royally.

"Anyway, you're off the hook as far as I can tell. No one really knows what you did. Maybe you owe me one?" Daniel asks.

By now, my eyes are brimming with tears. This is not good. He knows I dropped the ball, to say the least. I hate that he's seen me being a lousy doctor. And what's worse, he's saving my ass. He's caught me before I've fallen. It could've gotten ugly for me. The AES attendings could have made it a very big deal, especially if she didn't pull through. Somehow, whatever has happened with the patient, Daniel has smoothed the whole situation over.

I'm ashamed, but what really sucks is, I should be grateful. It's just the kind of thing I could easily get hung out to dry for, but he is protecting me.

What am I supposed to do with that?

Daniel and I go back a long way, and our relationship is complicated. There was a time when I really could have called him my friend, back in our residency. But now, there is too much water under the bridge, and I don't know what to think of him anymore.

I don't know whether to pity Daniel or despise him. I just know that he always seems to need me to defer to him, to subordinate myself to him, and it's the need that drives me crazy. But I have to hand it to him: He did have my back this time. I turned away a Tylenol OD. She could've died, or needed a new liver, and I would've been responsible.

"Thank you, Daniel, really. I do owe you for that."

"Mmmm-hmmm," he gloats.

"How are we going to do this?" I ask, blowing my nose as I slump into a chair. "Lucy was our buffer."

I should have realized a lot of things before. Daniel and I were only united in our love for Lucy; we both knelt at her altar. With her gone, we have no church community anymore. I never appreciated how much she was keeping the peace between me and Daniel until she pulled out of the triangle. I never had to deal with him much until now, thanks to her. He and I are more alike than not, and I think Lucy knew this. I can't tolerate his faults because they are my own.

"I know, she *was* our buffer," he acknowledges, sighs, and sits down at his desk. "I don't know how we're going to do this. Go home," he says kindly.

L
ucy's secretary Loretta loved Lucy, but she was never a fan of Daniel, and she's not particularly interested in working for him now that he's the new boss. She is putting out feelers for a different position somewhere else in the hospital. One of Loretta's main tasks is to maintain the moonlighter scheduling. The bulk of her time is spent calling and emailing various psychiatry residents and attendings for hire, making sure there are enough bodies to staff the CPEP and the up-wards on the evenings, weekends, and holidays.

One Wednesday morning when I'm in the country, at the house that Jeremy and I had bought not long before, I get a call from Dr. MacKenzie asking me if I would be willing to take over the scheduling if Loretta leaves her post.

"Of course I will," I assure him. I assume this will be a temporary stopgap measure until her replacement is hired, and I'm happy to help out. I want MacKenzie to know that I'm a team player, and I'd do just about anything for Bellevue.

I create a folder of the monthly scheduling templates and compile a mass email list of all the moonlighters, adding their pager and office numbers to my PalmPilot. I assume if I am organized (which I am, bordering on neurotically obsessive), it won't be too much trouble to keep the moonlighters happily employed.

As the months progress, I realize I have made a horrible mistake. The scheduling not only takes up huge chunks of my time, it's always on my mind. I obsess over every unplugged hole. I call Daniel at home one night to let him know I cannot continue to do the moonlighting schedule. We have a ten-minute conversation about this and that, and then when I bring up the scheduling, he finally relents. "Just tell me the last date you're willing to do it so I can find your replacement."

I give him the most obvious line of demarcation in the medical calendar.

"July first. Fine. Can I go finish my steak now?" he asks, peeved.

Steak. July. The screen swirls. I flash back to the Fourth of July, nearly two years ago, when Lucy invited all the CPEP faculty out to her East Hampton house to see the fireworks. It was also the first weekend with Michelle on the scene. I never would have predicted the teddy-bear girl would become the boss's girlfriend, but that's just what happened. Shows you what I know. At least he doesn't have to share his steak tonight.

"I'm sorry, I didn't know you were eating dinner," I reply. "You should've told me when I called; we could've spoken another time." It's just like him to play the martyr, not bothering to mention that he has sat down to dinner until the end of our call.

So, July first comes and goes and yet, somehow, I am still doing the scheduling. No one can understand why an M.D. is assigned to take care of a secretary's job, and I can't help but feel it's punitive in some way. Daniel is punishing me, keeping me under his thumb with this assignment. I also assume the reason I am still doing it after our agreed-upon date is passive-aggressive on his part. He wants me to come begging to him again.

At the next faculty meeting, when I mention yet again that I am tired of doing the scheduling, Maxwell, one of the attendings turns to me and says, "That reminds me, I'm going on vacation next month. Can you find someone to work my shifts?"

I explode, first at Maxwell and then at Daniel.

"Well, it's just that you did volunteer for it. You told Dr. MacKenzie you'd take care of it. And you have more free time than most of us," explains Daniel.

"You have a new secretary already, why can't she do it?"

"Dr. MacKenzie feels it needs to be done by a physician."

I'm going to need to talk to MacKenzie about this. There's got to be another solution.

I just want things to go back to the way they were. I want Lucy back.

Another Saturday Night

Sometimes the cases I see hit close to home; tonight I decide to buy a man dinner. In all my years at Bellevue, I've never once bought a man dinner. I'll occasionally kick in a few bucks to get someone onto a bus or subway and out of my ER, but I've never paid for a meal.

A mild-mannered, anxious man dressed in a suit and tie walks into the CPEP. He is temporarily homeless and afraid of the shelters, and he has lost his medication. After I give him some medicine, rewrite his prescriptions, and discharge him, he asks, "Can I maybe just collect my thoughts in this waiting area for a little while?"

"Of course you can, sir," I answer kindly. I give the hospital police a knowing look, the kind that says *Let him hang out for a bit and then send him on his way,* and the cop winks and smiles. A few hours later, on my way to the coffee shop for some dinner, I see that the patient is still sitting in the nondetainable area. Though he is seated, he looks lost, unsure of where to go next.

"Sir, if you don't want to leave the hospital, you don't have to, but you really can't stay here too much longer. Sometimes the police will let you sleep in the waiting room of the medical ER. Do you want to do that?"

He looks up at me and nods nervously. "Would that be okay?"

"Sure, it's usually fine." I try to explain where the AES is, but decide to walk him over there instead. On the way over, I ask him, "Are you hungry? Have you eaten?"

"I haven't eaten in two days, actually, doctor."

I take him over to the waiting area, schmooze the HP to let him stay, and get him settled. "I'll be right back."

I go to the coffee shop and order myself the usual Caesar salad with salmon (try it if you're ever in town). The guys behind the counter are funny and friendly, as usual, and I am bathed in their warm, loving smiles. I add on a cheeseburger, fries, and a soda. It makes me feel good to bring it to him in his chair. He seems surprised, and sheepish about accepting the bags of food.

I think it's his suit and tie that did me in, and the fact that he is so genuine. No defenses about him, no lying, no bullshit. Just innocence and fear.

I go back to the CPEP and am greeted with a new EMS case. A manic lady pulled naked off her roof, ranting and raving (you will never see one without the other on the EMS paperwork) in a loud, rhyming stream-of-consciousness that is pure Americana. Bits and pieces of these United Altered States, snippets from ads, sound bites from CNN. "If it doesn't fit, you must acquit!" "You're soaking in it! Mild? More than just mild!" "They're magically delicious!" "Your mission if you choose to accept it . . . Accept the unacceptable!" She goes on and on, and I am impressed at the catalog of slogans and insights she has at her disposal. I order some medication for her and go inside.

"I got a live one for you," I say to the resident coming on. "Should be an easy admit."

Rita comes out of the clerk's office to tell me that a patient from upstairs has just jumped out of a window onto the pavement outside the hospital. The hospital police brought the patient to the AES, but the man is dead.

A short while later, Desmond, the star resident of his class who was the apple of Lucy's eye, comes down to the CPEP. He looks pale. He sort of fidgets around, looking like he needs to talk. I ask him what happened with the suicide. I know he's working upstairs tonight.

"A young Vietnamese guy on the neurology ward. He was in for pseudoseizures," Desmond begins. This means the patient is having some sort of episodes that look like seizures, but when the neurologists perform an EEG to detect the brain's electrical activity, the results aren't consistent with true seizures. Sometimes, people with epilepsy fake some of their seizures. Other times, there is no true seizure activity at all, the pseudoseizure is an elaborate ruse, a well-choreographed plea for help or attention. "He's got a pretty significant history of physical abuse. His father beats him, it looks like. I think the problem is that he was scheduled for discharge soon, and he was petrified about going back to live with him."

"Was he on a one-to-one?" I ask. This is the highest level of observation the hospital can provide. If a patient is suicidal, they are assigned a staff member to sit with them twenty-four hours a day to keep them from harming themselves.

"He was for a while. The consult service was following him. The nurses called me because the order was written by a psych resident doing a neuro rotation, not the consulting psychiatrist. I was on the phone with them giving the okay to restart the order."

"So you restarted it?" I ask.

"Five minutes before the guy jumped." This lets psychiatry off the hook to some extent, and we both know it, but there is no relief in Desmond's eyes.

"How did he get out the window?"

"There's some controversy over whether he smashed the window with an IV pole or whether he just hurled his body against it. But the window looks just like a body went through it."

"Like a cartoon?" I ask.

Desmond looks at me witheringly, pityingly, and walks away.

What the hell is the matter with me?

Desmond is the poster child for Karuna, the Buddhist concept of infinite compassion. We both want others' suffering to cease, and yet we go about it in completely different ways. Should I be more like Desmond, with his limitless undying love? My patients would be better off if I could stay opened up and available, giving and understanding, yet my remoteness resurfaces routinely in my work at the hospital. It is my protection, like a hazmat suit, and it's been effective, so it's hard for me to move beyond it, even though I'm trying.

When I started out in 1996, I was a single gal with a boyfriend, holding a weekend job with a lot of time to kill during the week. I was confrontational, oppositional—a tomboy. It was as if I was reliving my rebellious adolescence during my first few years at the hospital. Acting as though I was too jaded to be shocked by anything, I challenged the EMS drivers, *What else ya got?*

As the years went by, I added a private practice to the mix, seeing patients on Fridays in my Greenwich Village office. Then, a few more years in, I got married, bought a house in the country, had a baby. As my life got more complicated, I learned to compartmentalize.

These days, I keep four bags organized in my closet to help keep track of my many personae—harried Upper East Side mom, tony downtown psychopharmacologist, crunchy country Yuppie, boisterous Bellevue doc. I have my private practice briefcase, a brown leather attaché, very thin, neatly packed with selected patient charts, extra prescription pads, my office keys, and a portable memory chip to back up my PalmPilot. On the same hook in my closet is a black diaper backpack, for errands around the city with a kid in tow. Then there is the huge red backpack that I toss everything into for my days off at the country house, my sanctuary. Last is my Bellevue bag: a brown suede cylinder into which I stuff medical journals to catch up on, an extra scrub top in case I get puked on, my Bellevue ID and hospital keys. What also gets packed into that soft suede bag is my suit of armor, the one I've had since childhood, a thick shell to protect my soft underparts from being skewered.

But even with the cowboy act, there are still times when I get down off my high horse, when I really connect with a patient, allowing myself to truly, madly, deeply feel what he is feeling, or imagine what his life must be like. I do this tentatively, experimentally, to see how much I can take, peeking into a pained and lonely world. What it teaches me, first and foremost, is to appreciate all that I have in my life. I am a richer person because of Bellevue, having learned the value of what I own. It's corny, but I swear it's true. I feel tremendous gratitude when I leave Bellevue on Monday mornings, returning to the outside world—the sort of relief I used to feel when I dismounted my motorcycle after a harrowing ride. I count my blessings, taking nothing for granted—my legs, my sight, my health, my home. More than anything now, I cherish my sanity, knowing full well it can disappear in the wink of an eye, especially in the face of insurmountable stress. I have seen all that can go wrong, how faculties can crumble just as internal organs can betray.

I have seen other doctors "turn off" when they feel they can't help, or they're getting it wrong. When a clinician misses a diagnosis, or the patient is "failing their treatment," the unsuccessful doctor's disgrace turns quickly to derision and dismissiveness. *You don't have anything I can fix* turns into *You don't have anything wrong.* Or worse, if the patient is a woman and the doctor is a man: *It's all in your head; you're hysterical.* The clinician is afraid, plain and simple. Afraid of his impotence, of the enormity of his failure and what it means to all involved.

Heinz Kohut, a well-known psychoanalyst, writes about empathic failure, that the psychiatrist can't always succeed at knowing the patient's pain and helping to ease it. It is best to admit fallibility and apologize for the failure, but most physicians aren't schooled in the ways of humility. They want to help and heal, to cut, sew, and fix things, and they often get mean and angry if they can't, like a petulant child. At least I do.

The problem with CPEP is that it is no place for infinitely compassionate clinicians. It's just not set up for the bleeding hearts. Being malicious is never appropriate—Lord knows I've learned that from Mary—but it is crucial to maintain some distance. I've known that all along, and Desmond will figure that out too, soon enough. When he eventually gets a job as a CPEP attending, he will last only one year. He will be reluctant to T & R many patients, wanting to admit them and treat them all aggressively, preemptively, no matter how full we are upstairs. Desmond will learn over time that he cannot save everyone, he cannot fix everything, and he will leave CPEP early in the game, telling me he is "crispy," his term for burnout.

But not me. I will work for a few more years after Desmond comes and goes, my longevity a direct result of my hardened persona, my blessing and my curse.

I'm Only Sleeping

Please don't wake me."

Four words that have never come out of my mouth at Bellevue. When it is time for me to leave the CPEP and escape to my office and bed, around one or two in the morning, I always give the same spiel: "I wake up easy; I fall back asleep easy. You should have a low threshold for calling me. If you have a question, pick up the phone; that's what I get paid for. Just remember, there are no stupid questions . . . only stupid people." I pause here for a smile or a laugh, though I'm not always rewarded with one. "And also, this is very important, you CANNOT discharge anyone without my hearing the case."

When I was a resident, I felt it was important to let my attendings sleep. It was a matter of pride. I wanted to show them I was competent, capable of working all night on my own without their guidance. As an attending, I know that many of my residents likely feel the same way. However, as I am quick to remind them, it is *my* ass on the line if there is a problem with a discharged patient. I'll be the one named in a lawsuit if there is what we euphemistically call in medicine "a bad outcome," so it is not okay for them to fly solo on my watch.

"So," I conclude, "at some point during the night, call me and give me an update on the area, even if you're not discharging anyone. If I don't hear from you, I assume you're sleeping like I am."

I always let the residents know that I am available to them all night long, and this is why I take great offense at the faculty meeting when Daniel accuses me of telling the residents not to wake me up.

I immediately deny it and challenge him, "You find one person I said that to."

"The residents were complaining about you at their last meeting," he replies.

I know what he's talking about. A week before, one of the residents had called me to present a case and was giving me a long-winded, meandering case presentation. Since she had woken me up and I was trying not to fully engage, so I could get back to sleep more easily, I asked her to get to the point. She was offended that I had requested the "*Reader's Digest* version" of her presentation and processed it as a narcissistic injury, a blow to the ego. She complained at a residents' meeting where Daniel happened to be. (The irony is, she, too, eventually became a CPEP attending after her residency, and developed a reputation as one of the doctors who makes it clear she does not want to be woken during the night.)

Along with the accusation that I shut out the residents overnight, Daniel adds a few more complaints about me in front of my colleagues. I am working fewer hours than everyone else, and I am whining about doing the moonlighting schedule at every faculty meeting. He singles me out and pummels me verbally. I am defensive and angry as I loudly refute his accusations, and it is not pretty. One of the new attendings sits next to me, her mouth agape. As Daniel and I run out of steam, and the faculty meeting winds down, I notice an interesting coincidence. At this particular meeting when Daniel has chosen to chew me out, his adoring girlfriend, Michelle, and his henchman, Dave, are nowhere in sight. There are many subordinates, but no senior faculty aside from Daniel and me. He has picked a good time to get on my case, making sure his compatriots aren't there to see the carnage, lest it sully their image of him.

After the meeting, I go straight to Dr. MacKenzie's office to complain about Daniel, his treatment of me, and all of his recent behavior. I may as well be running to my father to complain that my brother is teasing me: *Danny's picking on me! He started it!* I am fuming, rehearsing in my head the litany as I march through the bustling hallways to the other side of the hospital, dodging women wearing saris, men in dashikis, other men in heavy black suits and yarmulkes, their hair curled in front of their ears. I swim upstream toward the entrance as hundreds of Bellevue staffers work their way into the building.

The hallway that leads from the outside world to the inner workings of the hospital has the same brisk, bustling feeling as Grand Central Station, but the mix of nationalities is reminiscent of Ellis Island. (The welcome sign for the pediatric emergency room is written in seventeen languages, painted above and alongside the double doors.) Families come in to visit their loved ones; patients arrive for their clinic appointments; concerned mothers, their sick children wrapped in blankets, search for a doctor. I walk in silence, scanning each face, passing the wheelchairs stacked and chained in the corner. (The panhandlers steal them so that they can sit in them and appear crippled, to make their time spent on the corners more lucrative.)

Dodging the bodies, I am lost in thought. It's not just that Daniel likes to tear me a new one, he likes to do it in front of an audience. Anal sadist exhibitionist. This is how I have described him to Mary.

I stop mid-stride as I stumble upon a startling revelation: I wonder if that's how Mary thinks of *me*? Maybe she thinks I'm the sadistic one and I project all my demons onto Daniel. Is it possible that he's not really the problem, that it's all just projected self-hatred?

Jesus.

I resume walking, my hand on my forehead. *I can't waver like this when I present my case to MacKenzie,* I say to myself. I have to acknowledge to myself that Lucy's death has further complicated my perceptions of Daniel. I know he was a better friend to Lucy in the end than I was. He sat by her bedside in that hospital, not me; he was fiercely loyal to her, and he loved her as I did. He worked by her side five days a week while I only schmoozed with her on Monday mornings before I went home for the week. In truth, Daniel got a bigger piece of her than I did, and I was jealous. He's a good doctor, hardworking and generous to a fault. He is charcoal gray, not black, *but I can't paint him as such when I complain to MacKenzie, who can smell ambivalence, who's a shrink like you, don't forget,* I ramble on in my interior monologue. And don't cry. You have to learn that it's okay to be angry. Women at work are always letting their anger make them cry, especially in front of a supervisor. Bosses at work are usually processed as father figures. Don't make this about your father.

I take a deep breath outside of MacKenzie's office. *He is not my fa-ther,* I say to myself emphatically, knocking on his door.

"Daniel is totally out of control," I hit the ground running, barely letting my ass hit the seat before I begin my screed. "He is being a complete pig. First of all, at the faculty meeting two weeks ago, he makes a disgusting joke about ordering 'vagina au jus' at a restaurant." I make a face, to show I am repulsed by this ribaldry.

MacKenzie is impassive, silent. His fixed gaze and upturned face imply I should continue.

"I have as dirty a mind as the next guy, I'm sure you know, sir, and I can appreciate a good joke, but that was disgusting, misogynistic, and also—honestly—not particularly funny. Then, one Monday morning he says to me, in front of his secretary, 'You were much more fun to be around when you were pregnant with Molly. You should go home and get yourself knocked up again.' Do you believe that?"

I stop to see his reaction. Dr. MacKenzie cocks an eyebrow slightly, but doesn't look too taken aback. *Come on, man, at what point will you join me in my outrage?*

"And now this morning . . . he totally humiliates me in front of my colleagues, accusing me of being a slacker and telling the residents not to wake me up, which is completely bogus! I would never say that." I am steaming mad, lobster-red in the face, fighting back tears while I try to convey to Dr. MacKenzie what an impossible child Daniel is being, without sounding like one myself. I start to imagine a little girl running to her dad for support and coming up empty. This thought makes it infinitely harder to control the tightening in my throat.

Say something, Daddy!

I fill the silence with more whining, "Honestly, I really can't stand working for him. Under him is more like it. He insists on my subordination, and I have no respect for him anymore. And you know what happened to his hand, right?"

Daniel is wearing a cast on his arm. He punched the employee refrigerator in the nurses' station during a particularly dramatic exchange at a staff meeting. One of the psych techs was leaving the CPEP to go work upstairs, primarily, I believe, because of issues having to do with Daniel. Daniel had asked something at the staff meeting along the lines of "Who's with me?" and this particular tech had made a complaint, or implied that he wasn't on board and was abandoning ship. So Daniel growled and popped the fridge with his fist. There was a dent on that fridge for the longest time. Someone had circled it with a pen, as though to outline the evidence of Daniel's poor impulse control.

"I know, yes," Dr. MacKenzie utters casually. His first words of our meeting. He knows, but doesn't seem to care, that Daniel has assaulted an innocent kitchen appliance. A major appliance.

I was hoping for something more conspiratorial. Perhaps I had fantasies of us dishing the dirt about Daniel and his psychopathology, laughing about him, commiserating together. But MacKenzie remains stone-faced, giving me nothing to go on. He is my boss's boss, after all, and he's playing it close to the vest, as usual.

I pull myself together and get ready to leave the office. "All right, then . . . thanks for listening, I guess. I just needed to unload after this faculty meeting. He is really being an ass lately. One thing I can say, I don't think he's acting like a director should."

"Well, as you know, he is the acting director currently, and the administration is discussing whether to make that permanent."

"Obviously you know my vote," I stare into his eyes meaningfully as I stand up. "Thank you for your time, Dr. MacKenzie," I say faux-politely as I turn to head out the door.

"Julie," he says gently, motioning for me to sit again. "I liked what you had to say at Lucy's memorial, about how angry she was at having to die. I'm just wondering, how've you been feeling lately? I mean, don't you think it's possible you and Daniel are just angry that she's gone? And you're butting heads in her absence? Because your anger needs to go somewhere."

Ahh, the psychiatrist in him is emerging. He's good, actually. He has a smooth, caring delivery. I bet his patients like that. And he knows Daniel well enough to see what even I can see—that there is good and bad in him, as there is in all of us. Nonetheless, I persevere.

"It's more than that, I think," I join in on our new empathic level. "Lucy always said she couldn't trust him. That was something she spoke to me about a lot, when she first brought him down from upstairs. She thought he was smart, and he's good with the patients. He remembers cases, I'll give him that; he remembers people's stories. But there's something about Daniel that always bothered me." Here's my opening. Maybe we will conspiratorially get to dish and gossip after all. I can only speak my mind and see if he'll follow suit. "The line I usually use when I describe him is 'There's no *there* there.' He's all facade. That's what Lucy couldn't trust. She never knew what he was thinking, how he was feeling. There's something missing when you dig for the real him. You know, when I knew him in residency, he called himself Dan. Then he moves here and changes it to Daniel. Now, he's got the administration calling him Danny. He says it's his nom de guerre."

Dr. MacKenzie smiles widely at this.

"You're smiling," I say, "but I don't like that he sees it as a war, that it's him versus the administration. He spends most of our faculty meetings complaining about how hard it is being the boss, how he has to deal with all of these incompetents upstairs. I don't think it's appropriate for the rest of the faculty to hear how he has no respect for his superiors. How are we supposed to respect him, then?"

"Well, I appreciate your candor," says Dr. MacKenzie, wrapping up our meeting. "I'm not sure there's going to be any happy resolution here. Part of my job in this hospital is to try to satisfy everyone, address their complaints, and find compromises. What I end up doing, primarily, is spreading the misery evenly, thinly, so no one gets too much or too little. That's pretty much the best I can do."

"That sounds like a great job," I sympathize. I have an image of him as an aproned cake decorator smearing shit-brown frosting over a hospital-sized layer cake.

"I'll see what I can do," he promises.

"And that sounds like the parting words of a great administrator," I say as I leave. "I would appreciate your help on this one, Dr. MacKenzie. I've always thought of you as one of the good guys."

I've Just Seen a Face

On a Monday morning right before I sign out, I spy a man on a stretcher, lying asleep on his side. The word "Pussy" is tattooed on his right cheek. I am not sure who he is since he came in overnight while I was sleeping. During morning report, the resident signs him out as someone on triage who hasn't been seen by a doctor yet.

About a week later, I see the guy again as I walk by the coffee shop, on my way to have a meeting with Daniel and Dr. MacKenzie. I run into Daniel waiting for the elevator and mention it to him on the ride up, trying to break the uncomfortable silence. "That guy with the 'Pussy' face tattoo is back."

"It's an unfortunate word to be wearing, isn't it?" he asks, his manner arch, ironic. *An unfortunate word. Give me a break.* His irony only fuels my rage, but I control myself and join in on his level.

"I wonder if it's how he perceives himself, or if it's more a case of advertising what he's hoping to find," I offer.

We share the remaining time in the elevator in a stony silence; small talk and attempts at humor are useless. Dr. MacKenzie has asked us to come to his office to see if we can hash things out. I'm doubtful we can do more than hammer out the details of a détente.

MacKenzie opens the discussion with a bombshell.

"Daniel, Julie has made some serious accusations against you, regarding sexual harassment."

"No I didn't! I don't feel sexually harassed by you!" I squeal. "Hardly,"

I harrumph. "That is not what I said at all. I just told him about how you chewed me out at that faculty meeting. And how you told me I was a lot more fun when I was pregnant with Molly and I should just go home and get knocked up again. And about how you made that gross joke about vagina au jus." I stick that last bit in with pleasure, knowing it will infuriate him that I have shared his inane joke with his boss.

"Okay, not sexual harassment, per se, more like sexually inappropriate," Dr. MacKenzie calmly says. "Can we just agree that there will be no sexual comments, innuendos, or jokes in the workplace?"

"Of course," we both acquiesce. That's easy enough.

"Now, I understand you and Julie go back quite a ways, isn't that right, Daniel?"

"Yes, sir. We did our residency together," Daniel answers pleasantly. "I was, what, a year ahead of you?" He asks me as if he doesn't know damn well he was a year ahead of me. Like he doesn't remember doing a rotation together on the inpatient ward at Sinai, when I pissed him off because I stepped in as his patient visibly deteriorated. Hannah. It was over ten years ago and I can still remember her name. I couldn't stand by and do nothing when she was so obviously overmedicated, but it sure pissed him off that I broke the chain of command.

"That's right. We do go back a long way," I say simply. "But now can we please deal with this scheduling situation? With the moonlighters? It needs to go to someone else."

"Well, now, Daniel and I have been talking about this, Julie, and Daniel feels that it's appropriate for you to do this extra work because you're working less hours than the other attendings."

Fewer, I think to myself, but I dare not correct him. I also don't tell him how I'm not working any fewer hours than most of the other doctors. Most of us are logging in less than what is required to be considered full-time. "So why don't you just demote me to part-time?" I offer. "I've been working these hours since way before Daniel became my boss. All of a sudden I'm not working enough, so he thinks he can justify my doing the scheduling? That's absurd. Can I switch my status to part-time? Would that work?"

"Well, you changing to part-time is potentially a solution. Here's another suggestion I had, if you really don't want to do the scheduling anymore," he says, as he slides over a piece of paper to me. On it is a bunch of numbers, a chart of various hours and salaries. "You can either pick up some more hours and work another day during the week, or you can take a small cut in salary if you'd like to keep your current schedule."

"You've got to be kidding me." I can't believe this is happening. I look at the numbers. "You guys want me to take an eight-thousand-dollar pay cut? I've been working the same hours for years! I make one visit to your office to complain about Daniel being a pig and it costs me eight thousand bucks?"

"Now, that's not what's going on here, and I think you know that. If you take this new salary, you'd still be the highest-paid doctor at CPEP, based on hourly earnings, which is commensurate with your seniority."

"But I'd be making less money, doing the same job I've always done."

"This is your choice, Julie. You can keep doing the scheduling, you can pick up another day at CPEP, or you can take the pay cut."

"How long do I have to think about it?"

"How's a week? Is that enough time?"

I nod my head and get up to leave. My eyes are stinging with tears, and I have no desire to let Daniel see how upset I am. I'm sure he's grinning smugly, thinking he's won this round, which he truly has. He's got me right in my pocketbook, which hurts me more than anything.

"You understand that I am supporting a new family right now?" I remind Dr. MacKenzie. Emotional blackmail—it's worth a shot. "This pay cut couldn't have come at a worse time."

I leave the administrative suite, ride the elevator down to the lobby, and go to my office to get my things. I feel like I've been betrayed. Punched in the stomach. By my dad.

It's Monday morning, and I can leave for the week. I have a few days to decide what to do, although I'm already pretty sure that I'm willing to part with eight thousand dollars a year if it means extricating myself from this ridiculous scheduling job. That's what my peace of mind is worth, "eight large," as they say on *The Sopranos*. I start to fantasize about hiring someone to get these guys whacked. It's gotta cost less than eight grand.

Six days later, Sunday night in CPEP, and who should appear again but the Pussy-face-tattoo-man. He arrives by ambulance, after calling 911 from a pay phone on a street corner.

"Patient reports hearing voices telling him to kill himself, and he has taken two Tylenol number threes and one Vicodin in what he is calling a suicide attempt," EMS tells me.

"That sounds like a pretty good way to get high, but a lame-ass way to kill yourself," I say to the ambulance drivers. They laugh, as they always do. They're the only ones more cynical than we are, I think. Or maybe it's the cops.

I've seen this guy hanging around CPEP and the Bellevue lobby way too often in the past couple of weeks. Plus, now I associate him with Daniel, which is probably why I make the taunting comment right in front of him. He symbolizes all that is wrong with my job at the moment, and he must pay. My malingering radar is up pretty high after hearing a story like that, so there's no way he's going to be able to get past me tonight. *I know guys like this,* I think to myself. I already know his pants are on fire. It'll be tough for him to convince me otherwise. He is destined for the door.

"He's gotta go; we got way too many patients in the area," I say to Vera, the tall, thin, blond head nurse on tonight. "I've gotta clear the rack. Vera, you wanna join me in here for this guy and we'll try to bang it out together? I don't want him to get too comfortable here."

"The tattooed lady?" she jokes.

"Let's pretend we just can't see his face," I advise her.

We invite him into the triage room for a quick interview.

As he sits down across the table from us, he turns his head to the right, and I finally get to see the left side of his face. Up until now, I had only seen the right side, the "Pussy" side. His left cheek has a tattoo on it as well. "Licker" it says. Aha! Not just Pussy! Pussy Licker! This guy is advertising to all the ladies out there that he is available for their dining and dancing pleasure. Only, I guess it's not working so well, because here he is looking for a room at hotel Bellevue. I have to take a deep breath and try to maintain my composure before this man, with these words on his face.

Before I can even start the interview, he is already off and running with his laundry list of symptoms.

"I'm hearing voices to kill myself." He jumps right into the middle, no "Hello, how are you doing this evening?" I can't even get my fork out for the first question and he is already on his dessert.

"They're saying 'Why don't you just do it already?' and I haven't slept more than thirty or forty minutes a night for the past month. Also, I'm seeing my dead mother in front of me, saying 'Join me.'" He takes a breath to gather up speed for more, and I am nearly speechless. He is pulling out all the stops, and so early in the game. I've never seen anything like this, the impatient approach to convince me of insanity. And this last one, the "Join me," is a smart move on his part. I don't know if someone's been coaching him or if he just happened upon this symptom through trial and error at various ERs, but it's a doozy.

Identifiable auditory hallucinations are a more potent form of voices, a step above a murmuring mumble, "Kill. Kill." It is one thing to hear a voice if you don't know whose it is, or can't quite make out what it's saying. It is another thing entirely if the speaker in your mind is God or the Devil, or Jesus or your dead mother. Don't you usually do what your mother tells you? If you believe in it, you're more likely to obey it, and that's when things can get dangerous.

When I'm speaking to someone who is psychotic, I poke around for a delusional framework surrounding the voices. How believable are they to the patient? Has he followed commands in the past? When I was a second-year med student at Temple, there was a patient who chewed off a few of his fingertips when he was in the isolation room on the inpatient ward. He heard a voice saying "Prove your worth. Prove your worth," over and over. He believed that this was the voice of Buddha, challenging him to demonstrate his devotion. This patient decided that biting off his fingertips would send a powerful message to Buddha, that he was a strong and worthy disciple. Because his auditory hallucinations had delusional content, they carried more weight and were more likely to influence his behavior.

So, this guy with his tattooed face is giving me the line about his dead mother saying "Join me." It's a sneaky, calculated move. I've only met one other malingerer who used this tactic. A Vietnam vet I got to know while I was working at the Bronx VA Hospital. That guy followed me down to Bellevue for a while after I left the VA, but he gave up because I wouldn't admit him once I got settled in my new digs. More important, he came into a lot of government money when he won some back-owed cash for a disability claim. The last time I saw him at Bellevue, we were talking investments—stocks and bonds versus real estate—so I knew I wouldn't be seeing him for a while. But before the money came through, he used to go from ER to ER, where he would report hearing his dead father's voice saying "Join me."

"Works like a charm," he told me. "I get admitted almost every time with that line. That, and I put an unloaded shell in my mouth and try to light a match to it. Freaks everybody right the fuck out," he beamed proudly.

I try a different line of questioning with Pussy Licker: "Why is it that I see you around the hospital so much?"

"I come to the clinic here to get my AIDS medicine," he tells me.

"So, I'm just curious. Why are you so rigorous about taking care of your health if you actually want to die?"

"Huh?" he asks. He does this a lot whenever I ask him a tough question. Any question, actually.

As the interview progresses, it sounds like this:

"Do you take any medications?"

"Huh?"

"Have you ever seen a psychiatrist before?"

"Huh?"

This starts to drive me insane, as it does Vera, who's sitting to my left in the triage room. We look at each other with raised eyebrows, lips pursed, sharing a moment as the "Huh"s start to amass in a pile on the table in front of us. Obviously, he's stalling while he tries to come up with a line, and his "Huh" is a way to buy him some time. It is an obvious "tell" that indicates that he doesn't have an honest answer for us. There's practically no point conducting the interview if all we're going to get is bullshit. Also, here's a man who claims he hasn't been sleeping for a month, hears voices, and sees visions (which he says are happening all day, every day, including right now), yet he doesn't look the least bit disheveled, distracted, internally stimulated, or preoccupied.

I know he is lying, Vera knows he is lying, and on some level, I do hope the Pussy Licker man himself knows he is lying. It's time to let him know that we aren't going to be able to gratify him tonight.

I break the news to him in a way that I hope will spare me too much hassle. "Sir, while you do have an excellent story, which many psychiatrists in the city would completely buy, you are unfortunate this evening for several reasons. One, I have been at this a long time and so I am not having any of it, and two, we have no beds to offer you tonight because we are full." I play this up. "If it were slower here tonight, I'd give you a place to sleep, but we just have no place to put you. Maybe you should try another hospital?" I cock my head coyly.

"You're not going to admit me?" he asks, incredulous.

"No, sir, I am not," I say as politely and deferentially as I can muster.

"Can I get a Xerox of my chart, then? And a copy of the ambulance call report sheet too? The dispatch lady from 911 said with that complaint, about hearing voices to kill myself and taking those pills, that I should be admitted anywhere in the city. She said to call her if I didn't get admitted."

In all my years, this is the first time a patient has asked me for a copy of the EMS sheet. I'm impressed. "That's a new one on me, man! A copy of the ACR? You are a piece of work!"

Then he tells me that while he was waiting to be seen in the nondetainable area, he was looking for a piece of metal to cut himself with. When that goes nowhere, he ups the ante. "You know, Doc, on top of the pay phone when I called 911, there was a razor. I shoulda just used that to cut myself."

The guy is starting to get desperate, laying on one veiled, and not-so-veiled, threat after another: He'll sue me and the hospital, he'll hurt himself as soon as he leaves here.

He finally asks me, "What happens to doctors like you who kick out patients and then they come back on a gurney?"

I tell him calmly, "It's never happened to me, so I don't know."

He stops talking then, and looks down at his lap. He has pulled his wallet out of his back pocket and placed it on his lap underneath the table. He reaches into his wallet, slowly. I am a bit panicky now, because he has mentioned a razor, so I don't know if he has one in the Velcro part of his wallet that he is peeling back. We are alone in the triage room with him, with no hospital police in sight, just Vera and I, and I've been pissing this guy off, as usual, though I was actually trying not to.

Live and don't learn, that's my motto.

I never do see what he takes out of his wallet, if anything, because he closes it back up, looks at me, and sighs heavily, angrily. He's got nothing. It was a ruse, just to scare me, which it did.

The last guy to open his Velcro wallet in front of me had a shard of mirror in it, and Mr. K, one of our more proactive psych techs, was on him in a heartbeat, swooping in from the side, wrapping his arms around the guy's torso. They both crashed to the floor. I remember thinking how chivalrous it was of Mr. K to take a fall for me, literally.

"Listen, do you want me to fill out the paperwork so you can get into a shelter?" I ask, as nicely as I can muster. It is a lousy consolation prize, and he knows it. He declines.

Vera escorts him out of the triage room, and he says to her, "I bet you would've admitted me if I punched that doctor."

"No, actually, we would've pressed charges and sent you to Rikers," she says with a saccharine smile.

Like the last guy who punched me, I want to add. But I keep that part to myself. No need to give him any encouragement. I go back into the nurses' station to fill out his paperwork, relieved that I have escaped another attack.

For now.

On Monday morning, I go to Dr. MacKenzie's office and tell him I'll take the pay cut. Life is short, and I need less bullshit in mine.

Here, There, and Everywhere

Tuesday morning, quarter of nine, and Jeremy and I are loading up the car to head to the house. I get Molly into her car seat and then put the AM radio on to hear a traffic update. A woman has called into the station claiming that a small plane's just hit one of the World Trade Center towers. She's looking out her window describing the smoke coming out of the tower, and now some other man is also calling in who's seen the plane hit. Their stories differ in terms of how big the plane is, but my assumption is that it's only a little twin-engine Cessna or something. Jeremy slams the trunk and gets into the passenger side.

"Some pilot just crashed into the World Trade Center," I tell Jeremy. We listen to the radio for the next hour and twenty minutes, as the story continues to unfold, more and more unbelievable. "I should be at Bellevue," I say repeatedly as we drive away from the city. "Whenever there's a disaster like this, I'm pretty sure we're all supposed to just report for work immediately."

"We're not turning around," he says.

Okay, I think. *We need to get Molly somewhere safe. She'll be safer outside of the city.* Maybe I'll just take the train back in, once she and Jeremy are settled at the house. They probably need me at CPEP. With the Pentagon attacked too, people must be losing it. The psychic fallout on the periphery of the explosions must be immense—people panicking, paranoid, in shock, traumatized.

When we finally get to the house, we're in time to see the second building collapse on CNN.

The phone rings, and I assume it is someone trying to track me down from the hospital, telling me I have to report for duty, but it is Spalding Gray. Being on the phone with Spalding is like having a front-row seat for a workshop of his next monologue. This time, however, he isn't regaling me with fascinating anecdotes, peppered with his neuroses. Now, there is something different, feverish in his delivery. He's unloading his mania onto me, his speech revealing the layers of his obsessions and delusions. It's still a monologue of sorts, but it's heaving with pain and pathology. He and Kathie have sold their house in Sag Harbor and they're moving a mile away to North Haven. Spalding has become obsessed with the move, convinced it is a cataclysmically bad decision. He regrets selling "the green house" and is wary of relocating. He rambles on about how unfit the new house is for habitation and how perfect the green house was for him and his children, and mostly about how he wants to turn around time, to undo the sale, the closing, all the things that can't be undone.

I try to sympathize with him. He's been through so much. A car accident in June has left him in a very bad state, physically and emotionally. He's been intensely depressed and has required multiple surgeries. He still can't walk very well. Maybe he's fixating on the house sale needing to be undone because it is more feasible than undoing the car accident. He's clearly connected them in his mind. He repeatedly reminds me about the coincidence of the names: The driver of the car that crashed into his in Ireland and the real estate broker who has sold his beloved green house share the same common Irish name, which he weaves into the tapestry of his obsession. It's all been too much for him to handle, and he seems to be unraveling.

I can barely get a word in edgewise until I ask him, "Spalding, have you turned on your TV today? Do you know what's going on?"

"What? What are you talking about?" he asks.

I hear Kathie in the background yelling at him that the World Trade towers have fallen.

"There are other things going on in the world, Spalding. Big things. Bigger even than your house, maybe. Go see what Kathie is talking about. Call me later, okay?"

I hang up and think for a moment about my compartmentalized life, the four bags in my closet that segregate Bellevue and Manhattan from my country house, my work days from my days off. My little plan is not exactly working today as Spalding's mania crashes through my barriers, as I putter around my house feeling like I should be at CPEP. And Spalding has breached some boundary too, crossing over the line from neurosis to outright mental illness. I need to call Kathie later to create a treatment plan. He needs more help than I'm comfortable providing.

I try to get Daniel on the phone to see if he wants me to come in, assuming it's total chaos at Bellevue by now. I spend the next thirty hours trying to phone in to work. All circuits are down. A fast busy signal with every number and every pager I try. We also can't email anyone; the dial-up keeps getting stuck at "authenticating."

It's not until Wednesday afternoon that I finally reach Daniel, who tells me that things are under control. They were prepared for five thousand casualties and evacuated most of the CPEP and the AES. They emergently discharged as many patients as possible from the inpatient wards, making space for surgery patients and burn victims. Stretchers were lined up on every wall, in the lobbies, and in the parking lots, but they only got something like two hundred patients all day. He is describing what I already know to be true. I have seen the empty stretchers on the television for the past two days. The wounded simply didn't arrive.

"We're fine here. Just come in this weekend," he tells me. I imagine he wants to run the show on his own; he wants the glory, the martyrdom. *Well, this is one big, juicy steak he won't have to share,* I think to myself. Of course, these malevolent thoughts are childish and irrational, triggered by all of my resentments toward Daniel, but the truth is, I'm relieved to be off the hook. I don't want to leave my family and our safe haven just yet. He is working—as I should be—and I'm more comfortable resenting him for it than feeling inadequate and guilty.

Tuesday and Wednesday, September 11 and 12, we have the most spectacularly beautiful weather at the house. I go kayaking and running. I sit on the grass with Molly and marvel at the warm wind, the stark blue sky with no airplanes, and the sparkling sunshine. Wednesday morning I bring home the *New York Times* from the A&P. The pictures are poignant and nauseating. I remain fixated on the horror of people in business suits jumping to their deaths. Those images are burned into my brain. Later, research on the people who witnessed the disaster will reveal that those who watched the bodies fall are the ones with the most severe symptoms of post-traumatic stress disorder.

We speak to Jeremy's sisters, one of whom lives in SoHo and is having to deal with constant sirens, National Guard blockades, and acrid smoke and fumes. We beg her to come up to the house, and eventually she takes the train with her husband and two kids. We spend the rest of the week hiking in the woods and eating big meals. The television is always on in the background. Rudy Giuliani has become "America's Mayor." It is his finest hour, and he is lucky. His term is coming to a close, and he was going to go out with a whimper, but the World Trade attacks are allowing him to go out with a bang, a hero by proxy.

Saturday night rolls around and we drive back into the city, no problem. I get Jeremy and Molly settled in the apartment before I take off for work. I park in the back lot, behind the hospital, which is now full of government vehicles. There are official-looking cars parked on every available surface behind the hospital, on the curbs, on the grass, everywhere. There is also a huge red, white, and blue school bus. One of the hospital policemen calls over to me, "Hey! You wanna meet Mike Piazza?" A bunch of the Mets and Yankees have come to Bellevue to visit the patients who are 9/11-related. I take a pass on Piazza, waving and smiling graciously.

I am eager to get into the hospital, curious if the CPEP will be busy or not, but it is unusually quiet—a ghost town in a ghost city. I take sign-out and learn we have only five people in the area, a ridiculously small number for CPEP. I can't imagine why, the weekend after the towers collapsed, we would have such a low census. The calm after the storm?

I see one interesting case, a man from Iowa, in the middle of a manic episode, who felt that he needed to be at "ground hero" to assist the excavation. He took a bus across the country, went straight to the financial district, and got pulled out of a restricted area where he had commandeered a backhoe.

"They needed my help," he explains to me.

After I do his admission paperwork, I go for a walk to find the Wall of Prayer out front; I've been seeing it on television all week, and I want a look for myself. As I pass through the AES triage area, I see cases of water bottles and boxes of food on the stretchers. There are fresh fruit, chips, sodas, and tons of brown bags filled with sandwiches, snacks, and juice boxes. "You Are A Hero!" is written on one bag. "God Bless You! God Bless America!" is written on another. No hero, I nevertheless grab an apple and head for the front entrance.

A navy blue billboard has surrounded the old parking garage for the past few months while some construction was going on; it is now covered with laminated posters. Each poster, in large handwritten letters, says "MISSING" across the top. They all have pictures of World Trade Center employees, or Port Authority police officers, or firefighters, EMS, or NYPD. Every one of these pictures features a missing person who is not just smiling, but beaming. They are holding balloons, celebrating their child's birthday or christening, or dressed to the nines for their prom or wedding. They are on their honeymoons in front of sunsets on beaches; they're holding new babies. One of the close-ups is of an older man with two small hands, one on either side of his face. Below it is the wide-angle shot, with his grandson on his shoulders, leaning over his head and nestling his cheeks.

"The missing" are of every race and age. They have birthmarks, piercings, and tattoos—we know because they are carefully enumerated as identifiers on the flyers—along with which floor of which tower they were last seen or heard from. The wall is covered with these posters, and on the ground below them are rows of candles and mounds of flowers lining the entire periphery of the blue billboards. People are loitering around the Wall of Prayer, and there are several television crews with bright lights and bulky cameras. Some Bellevue staff are waiting in line to talk to the reporters, and those still hoping to find lost loved ones are being interviewed as well.

I make my way up First Avenue, over to the city medical examiner's office next door, where they've set up a huge outdoor makeshift morgue. Electric generators are running enormous stacks of lights, spaced along the cross street between First Avenue and the FDR expressway. It's ten o'clock at night, but it is bright white in the alley between Bellevue and the medical examiner's office, and everywhere there are empty stretchers. Hundreds of people in police uniforms or disposable scrubs are milling about. The process of sifting through the remains, transported to the ME site in refrigerated trucks, has begun. But they must be between deliveries, because no one is working. The Red Cross and

Salvation Army have set up comfort stations for the workers, and there is food everywhere. Granola bars and cereal bars being promoted by General Mills or Kellogg's are stacked up in boxes. There are bags of ice, cases of spring water, and hundreds of doughnuts. There are shelters all over the city that could make good use of these handouts, and I hope they will at least get the leftovers in a day or two.

Entering the hospital through the ambulance bay, I make my way back to CPEP again, but they have little need for me tonight. And then who should appear but Mary Ann DeLeo? I haven't seen her since she wrapped up filming the HBO Bellevue documentary.

"Hey, Julie!" she says, giving me a hug. "You want to help me find the fire marshal?" Somehow, she has set up a session to perform Reiki on him. I knew she was into yoga, but I didn't realize she knew how to perform this special massage, which I think of as a "psychic rubdown." She needs to meet him at the morgue, and she wants me to take her there. Mary Ann and I head out the back exit of the hospital.

There is another Wall of Prayer, this one behind the hospital, and it is for NYPD, NYFD, and EMS workers specifically. It starts to sink in a little more what has been going on these past five days that I have been out of the city. I start to think about all the EMS workers I know, the cops I've met over the years, and then I remember the Port Authority police. They bring us patients too, from the bus terminal, and it occurs to me how much they're just like the hospital police I hang out with every weekend. I worry about how many kids lost their parents this week, and that gets me worrying about the ultimate pain, losing Molly. It's a trip my mind will take again and again in the coming months, until I can train it not to go down that path.

Mary Ann and I walk right through the elaborate, two-tiered security system the state police have set up around the medical examiner's tent. The second pair of cops must have figured the first ones had already done their job, but we slipped right by the first pair easily.

"We must look like pathologists," I say to Mary Ann.

Everyone is just hanging around, eating the free snacks, hovering over the still-empty stretchers.

Mary Ann tells a receptionist in the ME building that she is there to see the fire marshal. In a few minutes, he ambles down the stairs with a colleague. These guys haven't slept in days, and it shows. They've lost scores of men; whole firehouses have been wiped out, and these two look pretty fried. I have offered Mary Ann the use of my office with its queen-sized bed to work her magic. No one will be disturbed there. When I finally go to bed some time after midnight, Mary Ann is finishing up with the second guy. He says he feels amazing. He can't quite understand what she's just done, but he's recharged and ready to go back to work, and he looks a lot better. I climb into my bed, where the fire marshal got just his aura tuned up, and I don't know quite what to think about my night. It takes me a lot longer to fall asleep than usual. I keep picturing the empty stretchers beneath the powerful lights, matching the faces from the flyers with the missing bodies.

On Monday morning, I'm done with my slow weekend and I decide to get my nails done. I haven't had a manicure in months, and my cuticles are bitten raw. Just like with the patients, I can always tell how I'm doing by looking at my nails. I'm not doing too great.

On the way into the salon, I stare at the headlines on the news rack outside the door. The *Daily News* front page has a grid of photos, maybe fifteen by fifteen, faces of police officers, firefighters, and ambulance drivers who are now dead. I think of all the wives who've lost their husbands, the children aching for their fathers. When the manicurist begins to rub my hands, massaging in the lotion, I start to cry and find that I can't stop. I put my head down so she won't see, but she does.

"What happen? You have fight with boyfriend?" she asks kindly.

I can't answer right away, just shaking my head as the tears fall down my cheeks. "They're all dead," I choke out.

"Oh . . . yes. Many dead, yes."

I am nearly a week late in my mourning and she is caught off balance, back to business as usual, assuming I'm upset about a romance gone awry. It is only when I am being pampered, massaged, and taken care of for a moment that I finally let my guard down enough to feel the pain of what has happened, the dismay at the destruction, the horror, the lives taken, the lives forever altered.

I am having a delayed reaction because, quite simply, I was out of town. It was a unifying event for all who were there that Tuesday, the Pearl Harbor for our generation. The city huddled together, under an attack now central to our history and culture. I am feeling like an outsider in my own city. I hate that I wasn't there to help, to comfort the refugees, the wounded, and the grieving.

When we have our next faculty meeting, I apologize to my colleagues, feeling the gulf between us.

"I'm sorry I wasn't here. I called Daniel and he said not to come in. . . ." I trail off. What is unspoken is that his words were enough for me. I know that other people wouldn't have called; they would've just shown up. Even Maxwell, who worked Monday night, came back in on Tuesday morning, explaining to me, "I just couldn't stay away." Like the man from Iowa with the backhoe, he felt he was needed.

The bomb goes off and initially we all scatter, fearing for our lives, but then some of us race back to ground zero to help in whatever way we can. There's a reason they were calling it "ground hero." I used to be one of those people.

Maxwell couldn't stay away, but I did, slipping into my role as mother and caretaker, not warrior, savior. What I couldn't fully communicate beyond my weakly conveyed regret and guilt at the staff meeting, was that although I was sheltered from harm, on some level I felt that I was cheated out of something potent and defining by not being in the city on 9/11. The world would forever be divided into before that sunny Tuesday morning, and after.

I didn't realize then that the psychic fallout would last for years. I would have a chance to help clean up after all.

Don't Let Me Down

It is Sunday morning, two months after 9/11, just before sign-out. I'm reviewing and signing charts from the night before, and taking orders for a coffee-shop run.

"EMS is here," yells lovely Rita from inside her glassed-in cage.

I go to see what they've brought me, and more important, which EMS workers have come. Since 9/11, every time EMS walks in, I am eager to see which of my pals is still in the game. I haven't seen some of my favorites yet, and that makes me nervous about their fate.

This time, it's one of the gals I've been waiting to see. There are certain EMS workers who stand out. This one, with her glitter nail polish and dyed magenta hair is quirky, sassy. She always reminds me of my sister in LA. She looks and talks like her, and they both paint their nails outrageous colors.

"I was wondering if you were alive!" I confess to her as I give her a bear hug. I ask her how it was, and if she was there, and she tells me this story:

"I was with my partner. We had just dropped off someone here at Bellevue and we heard that a helicopter crashed into one of the towers, or maybe it was a private jet, no one seemed to know for sure, but all hell was breaking loose in the ambulance bay. The staff went to DEFCON 5, and started lining up stretchers, paging for extra help to come down to the ER. So my partner says, 'You wanna go?' and I'm like,

'Why not? I got one more month till my pension.' And he said, 'You might as well go out with a bang.'

"So we drove down toward World Trade and all these other EMS rigs were heading downtown too, but everyone on foot was walking the other way. We set up right where we did back in '93, when it got bombed, remember? The second plane had hit by now and it was total panic. A free-for-all.

"After the first tower collapsed, debris was flying everywhere. The parked cars on the street were exploding. The building right next to us exploded and hot air was coming out of the lobby. I was getting thrown around by the air blasts, by the debris raining down, and then when the second tower collapsed I got hit with something on fire. My coat caught fire, and then my hair. If I had had anything like gel or mousse in my hair, I think my whole head would've lit up. I started running, and people were yelling at me, 'Stop, drop, and roll!' and I was like 'Fuck that!' and I just kept running. I noticed my shoelaces were on fire—not my shoes, 'cause they're leather—just my laces."

We both look down at her shoes.

"So I got scars from the burns on my back now, and my hair's a lot shorter, right? But I'm okay." She shrugs as she finishes her story, as if it were a recap of something a bit less life-threatening, say a trip to the corner store.

"Well, thank God you're all right," I say to her, sounding like a worried mother in a soap opera.

"Seriously. So, I went back there a coupla weeks ago and drove to the spot where we had set the rig up, y'know? And then over to the place I ran to? I can't believe it. I have no memory of running that far. I mean, I'm not in the best shape, right? I'm overweight, I smoke. Sixteen blocks like it was nothing."

I ask her how she's feeling now, if she's anxious or easily startled, or if she's had any insomnia or nightmares, doing a not-so-subtle screen for post-traumatic stress disorder. "Did you lose many friends down there?" I probe.

She gets a little teary as she counts them off on her fingers. "My best friend of ten years, on the subway, underground. A slew of EMS friends, a brother-in-law . . ."

"Well, I'm just glad you're still alive," I tell her again. "I've been waiting for you to come around. I still don't know who's dead and who's not. I just keep working every weekend, waiting to reconnect with all my old EMS pals, hoping they're okay. I guess I'll just hang here and wait until each one eventually checks back into CPEP with their crazy patients, so I can give them a hug like I gave you." I pause. "Or else I'm going to realize over time that they'll never come my way again."

Our town of eight million has been traumatized, and we are all still reeling from the blow. It's not just the city workers who are having trouble putting the pieces back together. We are all shaken. And there has been an interesting response by the medical community, an uptick in prescribing antianxiety medication and sleeping pills.

There was a time, when I first opened my private practice in 1996, when I had to leave a few minutes at the end of the initial interview for "the talk." I had to assure my new patient that it was okay to take psychiatric medications, that the pills were going to help. I had to sell my patients on the idea that there is no stigma to psychotropics.

Those days are gone.

My new private practice patients come to me with an agenda. Their friend, cousin, or dental hygienist is on this or that drug and they hear good things. They've seen the ads with the butterflies, or the smiling people on horseback. They remember particular brands from the women's magazines, and they have a few questions. But it's not *if* they should take medications, it's only a question of which one. Nearly everyone who comes into my office is assuming they'll leave with a prescription in hand. There is no longer any cajoling necessary.

Yes, the psychopharmacology business is booming since 9/11. After the twin towers fell, it was as if everyone suddenly had permission to medicate themselves: businessmen who were downtown and saw the bodies fall, mothers who were across town and didn't know where their children were, firefighters who lost their buddies. They came to my office fearful, dazed. They needed something to calm their nerves, to help them to make sense of it all, and so did everyone they knew.

The level of ambient hyper-vigilance in NYC has never really settled back to zero. After the planes hit, there was still anthrax, Afghanistan, Iraq, and al Qaeda to deal with. No one felt safe enough, or entirely sure about the future. Xanax and Klonipin are still flying off the shelves. As more physicians prescribe these psychic pain relievers, the trend is gathering speed, reaching a critical mass. Eventually, everyone will know someone who is taking *something* to help them relax, or sleep, or smile.

The fear instilled by the terrorists that day has insidiously grown and metastasized so that we barely register its presence. It has become the new norm. We are used to being reminded on the subway to "remain alert and have a safe day" and to being informed that our backpacks may be checked for weapons of mass destruction. Armed National Guardsmen are stationed at Grand Central Station in pairs, but we think nothing of it. Maybe that's partly due to all the antidepressants and antianxiety meds so many New Yorkers are taking now.

Across the Universe

Frequent flyers are the patients whom the staff sees over and over again at CPEP. I will sometimes joke about a patient being a gold-card level frequent flyer, or maybe platinum, to differentiate just how often we see them. The most common reason for recidivism is alcoholism or drug addiction. These patients walk into Bellevue, or are brought in by EMS, and they are completely drunk, high, or both, stumbling, disorganized, and occasionally aggressive. There's no safe place for them in the medical ER. They don't necessarily have an acute medical problem, and they tend to be belligerent and disruptive, so CPEP takes the transfer, sedating and housing them. I consider it a favor for AES more than anything else.

Usually, we don't get to do a full interview until the morning, when they're hungover and miserable. They typically want to leave the hospital, so they can get out there and do it all over again. Sometimes I will talk them into getting a detox bed upstairs, but more often than not there is no convincing them, no getting between them and their next fix, or their first drink of the day. So I step aside and let them leave. I let it go and move on, knowing they'll be back if their problems get bad enough.

Isaac Jackson, a frequent flyer, is a hulking menace of a guy. He's a meaty, tattooed thug who has taken a liking to PCP over the years. This, in and of itself, is unusual. The average Joe who tries PCP once never goes back for seconds. For most people, it is an unpleasant experience, unless you have a miniscule amount. It is common to become paranoid, thinking everything is a secret message for you to decode, that everyone is speaking a language you are not privy to. If you manage to smoke only a little, you may feel spacey, separated from your body, like you are floating on a cloud. But this is rare. More likely, you will become exquisitely fearful, which can turn on a dime to rage, if your paranoia can find a target.

Isaac typically comes into Bellevue angry, shouting racial slurs, threatening everyone within earshot with bodily mayhem. He requires heroic amounts of sedation—not for the faint of heart. I've had the pleasure of seeing him in these agitated states on more than one occasion, and I've learned just what combination of medications are required to tranquilize him. But this time, when he gets to the CPEP, he is all smiles and I barely recognize him. Only his tattoos assure me that it's the same guy. He's high on something, that's for sure. EMS tells me he was picked up after he refused to leave a McDonald's. The Ambulance Call Report lists Ecstasy as the likely intoxicant. I am intrigued. This is not his drug of choice, and he is out of his league, and in some respects, into mine. My Ecstasy book got published a few months ago; his timing is perfect.

"Isaac, what have you gotten yourself into now?" I ask, getting closer to him than I ever dared before.

"I'm high, Doc. I feel good. Don't mess with my trip."

"I wouldn't dream of it, darlin'," I assure him. I find myself sounding more like Lucy sometimes. Her Southern drawl always seemed to make everyone feel better.

Isaac's pupils are dilated. "Looks like you managed to find some good stuff. Let's you and me have a little talk."

Ecstasy, the popular name for MDMA (methylene-dioxy-methamphetamine), has a fascinating history. Before it became a recreational drug, taken at clubs or all-night underground parties called raves, it was used by psychiatrists and therapists. They would administer MDMA to their patients to help the therapy go deeper, faster. Feeling serene and loving, the patients could open themselves more fully to the process of digging up painful memories of physical and psychic trauma. MDMA gained a reputation among these psychiatrists as a powerful catalyst, helping patients to get to the heart of their problems. I interviewed many therapists for my book and was convinced they were on to something big before it became illegal.

Now I can see for myself just how well it works. I finally have Isaac where I want him. For the first time, he is actually going to receive some treatment in the CPEP instead of just being tied up and put down for the night. He and I are going to go spelunking inside his dark cave to see if we can't figure out what is making him tick like a time bomb. I'm excited, as if staring across the Grand Canyon, about to do an Evel Knievel on my motorcycle. I take him into the triage room without a nurse.

"Do you want some water? Are you thirsty?" I offer. It's important to stay hydrated with Ecstasy, though excess water retention can cause a lot of medical problems during MDMA intoxication.

"Yeah, Doc. That'd be great." The water will feel wonderful to him, which will help to align us. He will have good feelings for me if I help him to feel good.

"Isaac," I begin, "I'm glad I can talk to you today. You usually come in here pretty pissed off. You're all riled up and it's hard to talk to you much."

"I know, Doc. I'm mad as hell most of the time. I'm mad at the world." He pauses for a minute, looking up at the ceiling. "It's like I'm stuck."

"Why do you think that is? You must know that it makes it hard for us to help you, when you scare us away."

"Yeah. I guess so. But I keep ending up back here, don't I?"

"I think part of you really is asking for help. Screaming out for help, actually. Does that make sense to you? It reminds me of a little boy trapped in his crib, screaming bloody murder for his mother."

He stares at me, blankly. His mouth hangs open, but he says nothing. Am I going down the wrong path already? I'm losing him, and I know I don't have much time. Ecstasy doesn't last for more than three or four hours, and I have no idea how long he's been high. I decide to go for the gold. Most patients with a diagnosis of antisocial personality disorder have had horrendous childhoods. They were abused physically, sexually, psychologically. They weren't born monsters, they were raised by monsters.

"What did they do to you, Isaac, when you were younger? Who hurt you? Can you tell me what happened?"

"They hurt me bad, Doc. They hurt me bad and I'm mad as hell about it. They shouldn't live with what they done to me!" He is shouting now. Spit is flying out of his mouth, and the hospital police are star-ing into the windowed triage room to see if I need help. I wave them off, and I make a point of making sure Isaac sees me waving them away. I want him to know I'm not afraid, that I trust him, and hopefully he'll feel that he can trust me, too.

"What happened? Can you remember what happened?"

"They beat me. A lot. They beat me all the damn time!" he yells. Then he locks eyes with me and tells me quietly, "And I got raped. I was just a kid. I got fucked, Doc. I got fucked up the ass by my own family. How fucked up is that?" His face reddens, scrunches up, and he is sob-bing. "Why did they do that to me? Why did they hurt me? I didn't hurt them."

I wait. I make myself shut up and wait. I know it is important for him to vent, to have a catharsis, but I also know it will only do half the job. I want to try to have a more complete therapeutic interaction with him, and I try to stay focused. I'm not used to this sort of thing happening in the CPEP. I'm a lot more comfortable with keeping everything surfacey and light. A huge, angry man has broken down and is crying in the tri-age area. HP has probably never seen anything like this either.

"I hate that they did that to me. They fucked up my life. And now I hate everyone and everything."

"Even yourself?" I ask.

"Even myself."

He is doing a great job, getting exactly to the place where he needs to be. I plow ahead.

"I know it's horrible. They should never have hurt you. You didn't deserve that. No one deserves to be hurt by anyone, least of all their own family," I say.

"I didn't even do anything!" he yells.

"I know you didn't, Isaac. I hear you." I am trying to let him know that I get it, so we can move on to the next step. "And I see you're angry, Isaac. Every time I've seen you, you've always been angry. But I want to tell you something. Listen to me. Look at me." I pause. He lifts his head up from his arms, folded on top of the triage desk. I wait until his tearstained face is engaged with mine. "They never should have done what they did. We both know that. It's completely fucked up. But we can't change what happened, right?"

"Right," he answers obediently.

"The only thing you can change is Now. Right now, you are doing their job for them. You are fucking yourself. You're finishing what they started. You have to stop it. You show them that you're better than that. You show them you can have a good life. You deserve better and you need to make sure you live better than you have been. You come in here over and over again, and you're high on PCP, and you're drunk out of your mind. And you get arrested, and you hurt people, and they hurt you. It's like a broken record, Isaac. All the pain, all the anger. You have to take the needle off the record. You need to make this stop. Do you think you can do that? You are fucking yourself, Isaac. You're taking up where they left off. You're letting them win. Can you stop it?"

He thinks about what I am saying. Should I have broken it down into smaller pieces?

"Can you let us help you to stop it?"

I have no idea if he's getting it. He is quiet, exhausted maybe. I sense the Ecstasy is leaving his system, and he is starting to shut down again, to close off the most exposed parts of himself. This is something he needs to do to survive, I know, but it is disheartening to watch it unfold in front of my eyes. I have the sense that he is reassembling his armor right in front of me. I'm not sure I got through to him. I don't know if it got into his head in time. He needs to rest, to process what has happened.

"They hurt me bad, Doc. They should die, what they did to me," he repeats.

"I know, Isaac. I know they hurt you. But you can't change that. You can only change *Now*. And the future, maybe. You can probably change that, too. You have to stop hurting yourself, Isaac. Don't keep doing their job. Don't keep fucking yourself." I'm purposely repeating simple phrases over and over again, hoping it will act like hypnosis, hoping some of it will sink in deeper, subconsciously, and make a difference in his life. But I can't tell if it's going to work anymore. I don't know if the MDMA has totally left his system or not.

"Do you want to sleep here tonight?" I offer, like he can crash at my pad. "I'll give you the best room in the house. You can think about what we talked about. Think about how you can make your life better, and in the morning, we'll talk some more, and you can meet with the social worker. You can come into the detox ward if you want. Let us help you, Isaac. Let us do our job; don't push us away this time."

I admit him to the EOU, to the largest room in the corner, which I like to think of as the VIP digs at CPEP. It *is* the best room in the house, though that's not saying much, seeing the rest of the house.

In the morning, after we've both slept, I go into his room to talk to him some more. I have a few minutes before rounds, and I want to see if he is still opened up at all, or if he has completely reverted to his intimidating old self. He is sitting on the floor, his back to the cot. His elbows are resting on bent knees. He looks up at me and smiles as I enter.

"Good morning, there, chief," I begin. "How are you feeling?"

"I feel pretty good."

"Do you remember what we talked about last night?"

"Yeah. I remember. You said I'm finishing the job they started. But they should pay for what they did to me."

So it's a compromise, half my mantra, half his. It's a start. "Isaac, you're making everyone pay for what some people did to you. That doesn't make any sense. Not everyone is the enemy. You can't go through life scaring everybody, pushing everyone away. We're not all going to hurt you."

"I'm mad at what they did. I'm mad at the world."

Great, we're back to that again. I try a different tack. "Isaac, let me ask you this: Who loves you? Who do you love? Where can you go to get some love?"

"I got a girl in Texas. We have a daughter together."

"You're kidding me. You're a daddy?"

He grins sheepishly at me, and then I know where he belongs. And so does he. "I'm going to talk to the social worker this morning and we're going to try to figure out a way for you to get down there."

"That'd be good, Doc. I think that'd be good for me."

"I know that'd be good for you, Isaac. There's just one thing. There's a lot of PCP in Texas. It's called "fry" down there. You gotta stay away from it, you understand? It's not doing you any favors, that drug. It makes you too scary. No fry, Isaac. Go down to Texas and get yourself some love, but stop with the PCP, will ya? And stop getting loaded all the time. You hear me? Move on! You gotta fix up your life. Try to start over. Be a good daddy, why don't you?" We shake hands, solid, strong, and I leave his room feeling buoyant.

I go into morning rounds to report on the patients in the area. When I get to Isaac Jackson, and tell the whole story, I get a little choked up.

Daniel doesn't let it go, of course. "Doctor Holland, I've never seen you get so emotional about a patient. This one really got to you, huh?"

In front of everyone, he is making me feel like a sap. I give a mini-lecture on MDMA-assisted psychotherapy. I try to defend myself, the experience I had last night, but mostly I am worried about my patient. I am worried that in the cold light of morning, with the indifference of a new shift, Isaac will simply be grist for the mill. Packed up and shipped off like any other patient: He was high, he's cleared, get him out the door and on to the next patient. I explain, in more detail than I probably should, the content of our session the night before. I plead with the staff to spend extra time with him today, to treat him gently, and to follow up on the plan to get him to Texas. At the very least, get him a detox bed. Daniel moves rounds along dismissively, and I seethe.

I find out the next weekend that Mr. Jackson was discharged on Monday morning, hours after I left, with no real assistance from us. I am told that he "didn't want detox." It pisses me off that they didn't do as I asked. The paranoid, neurotic part of me can't help but think that Daniel personally made sure that Isaac was discharged without getting what I wanted for him, though Daniel assures me that they did spend extra time with him and it went nowhere.

After one more drunken CPEP visit several months later, Valerie does help him to get some bus-fare money wired from his girlfriend, and we never see him at Bellevue again. I like to think he's a Texan now, down there with his wife and daughter, and he is making up for lost time, making his life better, finally.

I won't follow up and call him. I learned that lesson years ago. I won't even do a search on his name in the computer to see if he's been to the AES. I'd rather just pretend that he's found a happy ending. It makes my job easier.

Don't Panic

The night starts out light on December 14, the day after my birthday. There are only a dozen people in the area and no one on triage.

I make the mistake of appreciating out loud the low census, and the superstitious nurses shoot me a look. Oops. Sure enough, in the next hour I've got four triages and nowhere to put them. There's a long-standing tradition in medicine of avoiding certain words in the ER. I waver between being superstitious and not, but there are definitely ER staff who deem it bad manners to mention certain words: "calm," "quiet," "dead." They think it's like baiting the gods to screw with us.

Superstition is akin to something that psychiatry calls "magical thinking," the belief in talismans, omens. It's normal in most people, and easy for me to see why. Twice now at Bellevue I have uttered the word "dead" as in, "Man, it's totally dead in here!" and the crowds came running. Five EMS deliveries in seven minutes once, moments after the evil word was uttered. Now I allow myself the occasional "slow" or "easy" but rarely will I say the word "quiet" and never, ever "dead." Mostly, it is safer to never comment on the activity level of the ER when you are on shift, though it's fun to utter a prohibited word as you're leaving. Then it's someone else's problem. Tonight, though, it's mine.

A pair of EMS guys, two of my favorite clowns, bring in a patient who's been to Bellevue before. The 911 call came from the Port Authority police reporting an overdose in the bathroom. Jesus Martinez, at thirty-four, has end-stage AIDS contracted from IV drug abuse. Years ago, he unknowingly infected his wife with the virus, and she has recently died. Somewhere around four-thirty in the afternoon, he shot a big load of heroin and cocaine in a bathroom stall at the bus station, hoping it would kill him. At nine p.m., he was found by a janitor. He had been passed out on the toilet for nearly five hours, and had a temporary sacral neuropathy. Basically, his legs had "fallen asleep" due to the compression on his buttocks, so he was unable to walk after my two EMS pals revived him.

They regale me with the details of their pick-up, telling me there was vomit, urine, and feces at the scene. Mr. Martinez's colostomy bag had become unhooked, leaking its contents all over the bathroom floor. They make some joke about a trifecta, and we all laugh. "It's the holy trinity of body fluids," I add.

When they bring him to Bellevue, the EMS drivers assume the patient will be accepted at the medical side of the ER since he is an overdose with an inability to walk, not to mention the end-stage AIDS and colostomy bag. But the AES nurse signed off on him and told EMS to bring him to us. When EMS presents the case to me, they encourage me to "bounce him back" to the AES, as if I need encouragement to get rid of this guy; the stench is impressing even my veteran nose. I roll the man down the hall to AES, looking for the attending. I'm hoping he'll be cool and just accept the triage, do me a favor, but it's a new attending I've never met. She's Polish, or Russian maybe, and about five months pregnant. She looks cute in her scrubs with her little belly, and it's hard to hate her, even though she examines the guy a bit, asks him "Where does it hurt?" about half a dozen times, and turfs him back to me.

"The overdose was six hours ago. He's fine. His feet have good pulses," she says to me.

The fetid stink from his feet hits me seconds after she takes off his shoes. "Have you had much trouble working in the ER during your first trimester?" I ask her. "I remember when I was pregnant with my daughter, I really had a heightened sense of smell, and also more of a gag reflex than usual. Are you doing okay?"

She smiles, and we have shared a moment; belonging to the same club and all that. Then it passes. We discuss briefly the fact that he can't walk right now, which is a new symptom for him. I know he's got a temporary syndrome from the compression of his sacrum, but I'm playing dumb, asking if he's paralyzed from a stroke or something, hoping she'll take him and do a head CT. She minimizes all his physical complaints, findings, and history, and is gently making it plain that she is still not signing the EMS sheet, not accepting the patient to her area.

"You're getting hit with triages even worse than I am tonight," I notice. It is a peace offering, my mentioning how busy she is, and she takes it as such. She smiles sweetly as I decide to do her a solid and take a hit for the pregnant doctor.

Back at CPEP, we wheel Mr. Martinez to the high-visibility area, right in front of the nurses' station. I know a little about this man, because he has been admitted to Bellevue a handful of times in the past. He had a well-known hospital roommate awhile back, maybe a year and a half ago. A man on 12 South—admitted after he cut off his penis and the Bellevue surgeons reattached it—had attempted to escape from the hospital. The man spent days, or perhaps weeks, meticulously cutting strips off his mattress and braiding them together to make a rope. Then, he somehow pried open a window and attempted to rappel himself down the side of the building. Needless to say, the makeshift rope broke, and he fell roughly ten stories to his death on the street outside the hospital.

Mr. Martinez was traumatized by this, as were many other patients on the ward. He somehow felt guilty about his roommate's death. But the real guilt that was driving his current behavior was that, in his eyes, he had killed his wife. His years of shooting drugs into his veins had left him with AIDS, and he infected the woman he loved before he knew he was ill. Since her death six months ago, he has made several attempts on his life.

Between the overpowering foot smell and his burst colostomy bag, this guy needs a shower in the worst way. He's being nasty to the nurses, and irritable to the psych techs. He even spits at one of them.

"Go away!" he yells. "You babied me the last time I was in here, I don't want to be babied. Get away from me!" He lets Magil, the psych tech, change his colostomy bag, but then he starts complaining loudly about the pain he's having from his herpes zoster, aka shingles. AIDS patients, with their weakened immunity, often have herpes, which is a virus that lies dormant in the body waiting to be reignited when the patient's immune system lets its guard down. The virus hides in the nerve cells of the body, and when the herpes infection flourishes anew, it is immensely painful. And this is not a guy who suffers in silence.

I call the pregnant AES attending, wondering if there is any medication she specifically likes for the neuropathic pain of herpes, which is often treated differently from other kinds of pain. She tells me to give him Tylenol with codeine, or morphine. She knows he's shot heroin earlier today, but I go ahead and give him two Tylenol 3s, because his jaw is grinding away a mile a minute, which tells me the cocktail he shot up this afternoon must have had more cocaine in it than heroin. I write the order at ten thirty.

I've got five triages to deal with; I figure I better start in on the pile. As usual, I look for the easy T & Rs, people I can shoo out of the area with a minimum of paperwork. I leave the more complicated admissions for the resident.

The surefire T & R, one hundred percent of the time, is an arrested woman. If she's calm and not dangerous to herself and others, she goes back with the police to get arraigned. If she's insane or agitated, she goes to Elmhurst Hospital, which the city has designated for female forensic psych admissions, the counterpart to our 19 West, where the male cases are housed. I talk to the cop to see what the charges are, and why she was brought for psych clearance.

He shoots me a smile, and tells me, "You're gonna love this one, Doc. Assault with a deadly weapon. She attacked her husband with a huge plastic Santa Claus lawn ornament."

"'Tis the season!" I quip.

I speak to the arrested woman briefly, enough to establish that while she is schizophrenic and mad at her husband, she is not acutely psychotic, dangerous, hallucinating, or agitated. I send her out with the cop, who is impressed at how quickly his Bellevue detour has been resolved. He heads back to the station to book this woman, and I head back to the rack to pick up another case. I'm on a roll, so I pick up another chart, hoping for a second T & R. It is a woman brought in by EMS, accompanied by her brother, who tells me that he'll take her home with him after my evaluation, which is music to my ears. A family member willing to take responsibility for a patient means I don't have to fret so much about her disposition. The EMS sheet reports that her neighbor called 911. The patient was drunk, complaining on the phone to her neighbor about her children, making some veiled references to suicide, wishing she were dead.

I opt to interview her at what I call the picnic table, a sturdy metal version set up by the EOU rooms, under a TV to glance at in case I get bored during the interview. I strategically place her back to the television; *Saturday Night Live* is on. I spend about five minutes trying to cajole this woman into telling me what she said to her neighbor so I can document just how suicidal she sounded.

She is still a bit drunk, coyly skirting her exact words, and I feel myself getting frustrated because she wants to tell me the backstory. She tries repeatedly to unload her sorrows on me, about her children, her loneliness. What I really need is a direct quote for the chart: Exactly what did she threaten on the phone? Just as she's finally giving me the goods, I hear a frantic shout from one of the psych techs for me to come quickly. "Doctor Holland!"

"Julie. You better get over here," the resident adds, nervously.

Mr. Martinez is on the floor, and they're cutting away what looks like a long black shoelace from the stretcher, unwrapping it from around his neck. Once the string is removed, I can see its braided pattern embedded in his swollen neck. His face is mottled, purple and gray, and he is lying in an awkward position on the floor, his arms and legs arranged around his body at odd angles.

Bill, one of the psych techs, tells me, "He took off his hoodie tie and wrapped it around his neck."

With the other end tied to the railing of his stretcher, he has thrown himself off the edge of the gurney, hanging off the ground just enough to choke himself. I squat down to feel his wrist while Bill feels his neck for a pulse. I feel nothing, but Bill says, "I've got a pulse!"

Jesus is unresponsive—not talking, not breathing, as I rub his sternum and call his name. His colostomy bag has burst onto the floor, the maroon liquid spilling out into an ever-widening circle as the hospital police and techs put on some gloves and lift him onto his stretcher. I stand there frozen for a moment, then quickly decide to bring this guy to the medical ER.

"Let's get him to AES!" I yell. There is no way in hell I am running a code in the CPEP. It is such a rare event, and the staff, including me, is ill-prepared for it. He'll surely die that way. There is no time to second-guess myself, but it is a decision I will have to defend repeatedly in the days to come.

Bill and I push the stretcher out the door, as I yell at the patients to clear the way. We maneuver the stretcher out the CPEP doors, making sharp turns, right, then left, then left, then right, until we reach the straightaway down the long hallway to AES. There are multiple sets of double doors. Why are there so many doors? Dangling off the edge of the stretcher, his right foot hits one door jamb and then another, as we do our best to steer the less-than-agile gurney. We pull into the ambulance bay of the AES, as if we have a new EMS case for them.

"We need a doctor here!" I yell. (*A real doctor,* I think to myself. *Not a shrink. Someone who can save a life, like they do on television.*)

The chief resident runs over and directs us to wheel our patient into a spot by the door.

"He tried to hang himself from the stretcher," I tell him. "He has AIDS, a colostomy. He overdosed on heroin and cocaine earlier today."

The chief establishes that the patient isn't breathing and requires oxygen. While he bags the patient, putting an oxygen mask over his face, he asks me, "How long has he been down?" By this he means without oxygen, and it will be the question that runs through my mind repeatedly as the code progresses: *Why didn't I bag him while we were transporting him here?* I estimate a minute or two, taking into account the time it took us to speed him along the interminable corridor, but I can see the resident is skeptical.

A medical student begins compressions, and the chief says, "Real CPR, please," to the student. It must be a tradition, I think, flashing back to the chaotic scene at the codes when I was a medical student, when doing compressions seemed like the best role to play in a resuscitation. You feel you are being productive, you are doing something physically to help the patient, and it requires a minimum of know-how. But then the person running the code comments on your form, and the critique cuts you down to size, transforming you from the one who is saving the patient to the one who is killing the patient through your incompetence.

This chief has a way of making everyone feel incompetent though, and that's what he does to me when I make the huge mistake of mentioning to him, as he runs the code, that I had tried to get AES to take the triage and they refused.

"That's not helpful to me right now," he says testily, and I know he's right. I tell him the patient had two Tylenol 3s at around eleven o'clock, in addition to whatever heroin he injected six hours earlier, and recommend Narcan, an opiate blocker. It's the only useful piece of information I give him, and he begrudgingly orders Narcan, after making me wait and watch for a moment to see if he'll gratify me in this way.

One resident is attempting to get a sample of arterial blood from the patient's arm, another is putting a catheter into his penis, a third is putting an intravenous line into his neck. A nurse is filling syringes, serially—Epinephrine, Narcan, Epinephrine—stating the medication's name with solemn regard as she hands the needle to the chief.

The patient's heartbeat comes back after two rounds of "Epi"— a hormone similar to adrenaline—the stuff that is now surging through my veins and making my heart race, as I struggle to keep my hands out of my mouth and appear calm. The compressions cease, and the second-year resident tries for a second time to intubate the patient, craning the patient's chin toward the ceiling to see down his throat. She can't visualize the vocal cords, the landmarks to tell her she can proceed with the tube into his windpipe; because of the strangulation, there's too much swelling. The chief resident finally takes over, the savior, the martyr, to do the intubation like it's supposed to be done.

The pregnant attending ambles up next to me to watch her protégé run the code; I find it comforting to have her there. I imagine she's glad he was in my area, and not in hers, when he made the second attempt that day on his miserable, dwindling life.

"His pupils are blown," the chief tells the crowd. "Let's call respiratory."

I know what this means: Jesus Martinez is as good as dead.

He is placed on a respirator and admitted to the MICU, the medical intensive care unit, where they will likely try to contact the next of kin to discuss removing the respirator, assuming that he will stop breathing and die a natural death. Sometimes, however, these patients keep breathing on their own, and then we are left with what we call "a brain stem." The medulla, a major part of the brain stem—south of the cortex where the real feeling and thinking is orchestrated—is still functioning, reminding the lungs to breathe, instructing the heart to beat. During my neurosurgery rotation in medical school, the bulk of the patients on the inpatient wards were in this state. I would write notes that said VSS, CVSP: vital signs stable, chronic vegetative state persists.

And persists. If they don't get an infection, "brain stems" can live for a painfully long time, being fed through a tube into their stomachs. We would also sometimes refer to these patients as "rocks," immobile, immutable. We would come and go as we began and ended our rotations, but they never left the hospital.

I remember the afternoons on the neurosurgery wards, when the visiting families would come. The patients would lie there, dressed in their satiny sweat suits, breathing, blinking, hearts beating. Sometimes their eyes would move, a reflex of the lower brain centers; they seemed to follow their loved ones across the room, but a vegetative state is not fully alive, and the patient is not really "there." The eye movements often give the families false hope, which can complicate their decision to turn the patients into DNRs. It's hard for the families to understand that even though the eyes are open and moving, their loved ones are not truly seeing them.

So, Mr. Hernandez hasn't quite killed himself exactly. He has, thanks to our interventions, put himself into a medical purgatory. He's not alive, but he's not dead. His brain is functioning just enough to keep his heart beating, and our machines will keep his lungs filling with air, his blood oxygenated, his organs functional.

I come back to CPEP with the information that he is on a respirator in the MICU, which the staff takes as good news, that he has been saved, but they are wrong. He has basically killed himself on my watch, under our care, and it is only a matter of time and semantics separating him from actual death.

And now come the paperwork, the phone calls to the bosses, the questions, the revisions, the muted conversations, and the Monday-morning quarterbacking. I steel myself in preparation for the inevitable days ahead, when I will have to speak with the hospital administrators, the lawyers, my boss, his boss, and the boss above him, and the lawyers, the nursing supervisor, the next of kin, and the lawyers again.

MacKenzie calls me up at the house to ask me what happened, and I tell him everything I can remember. He tells me that on Thursday there will be what the Bellevue Department of Psychiatry calls a "Special Review." These reviews are supposed to be dispassionate dissections of what occurred, but inevitably they morph into a reaming of one or more parties.

Shortly afterwards, Daniel calls me to strategize for the inquisition.

He is upset when he finds out that I have already spoken to MacKenzie. He has a lot of specific recommendations for how best to answer the questions, and how to frame the situation in general. He jokes that I should cry during the Special Review. He figures if I look frazzled, they'll go easy on me.

At first I don't understand why he's calling to give me any advice. Why should he care if I take a fall? But then it occurs to me that it will reflect badly on him if there is any blame shouldered. He'd prefer the whole CPEP look innocent.

He reminds me to keep my responses to a minimum. I have a habit of overtalking and overanalyzing; in my most awkward situations, I get a case of verbal diarrhea.

When I see the AES chief resident who ran the code at a downtown restaurant a few weeks later, I apologize for doing just that.

"I should've just shut up after I gave you the bullet, but I was stressed and I kept talking. I shouldn't have said that you guys rejected the triage. It was right for you to respond the way you did," I tell him. Better for me to make peace with him, I figure. I may have to work with him again down the line.

He did, after all, prevent my patient from actually dying, and for that I am thankful. But our patient, he really wanted to die. I am sure of it. He would not be so grateful his plans were thwarted.

Carry That Weight

Dr. Henderson, the director of inpatient services, pulls me out of the up-wards conference room just before the Special Review begins. He squeezes my shoulder and murmurs, "Julie. No one thinks you did anything wrong. Go easy . . . go easy."

I am stymied, and offer no response. Sweltering in my most matronly sweater set, a sickening shade of pale green, I'm finding that it's only too easy to appear emotionally distraught. Daniel will be pleased that I am taking his advice.

I can't figure out if Henderson is telling me to relax because I have nothing to worry about, or if he is soothing me because he's afraid I will make a scene otherwise. I remember the phone conversation between us on that Saturday night, around one in the morning, shortly after the code. I started off on the offensive.

"Dr. Henderson, I know Bellevue," I began. "I've been here long enough to know that in these situations somebody usually takes a fall; someone is always left to twist in the wind. I just want to make it clear, sir, that 'somebody' is not going to be me." Maybe I even said it menacingly. I wanted him to know I wouldn't take any of this lying down. I wouldn't go quietly.

Everyone seems to be warning me not to sabotage myself at this meeting. They are all implying that my usual protection, my swagger, is my potential undoing. It certainly hobbled me at my oral boards, and I can't let that happen again.

The conference room is full of unit chiefs, department directors, and other high-level administrators sitting around a large, rectangular table. I choose my seat carefully, looking for allies. I am afraid for my job and for my reputation, and it's hard to figure out whom to align myself with. I sit between Daniel and MacKenzie.

Henderson calls the room to order and begins. "This is a very complicated case. And though it seems clear that this patient was marked"—he pauses for dramatic effect—"marked for death, this should not have occurred in our hospital."

I love that, marked for death. Henderson's got quite a flair for the dramatic. He asks to hear from the different specialties assembled around the table, and the director of nursing begins.

And we're off. There is some confusion about how many patients were in the area and how busy we were that night. I look over at Daniel questioningly, with terror on my face, and he does something cryptic but potentially communicative in its symbolism. He begins to draw on my Special Review handout—a schedule of who is to speak and in what order, with Mr. Hernandez's initials and medical record number at the top of the page. Is Daniel writing me a note? No, he draws a tic-tac-toe board and he puts an X in the bottom right-hand corner. He slides the paper toward me.

Tic-tac-toe. . . . Yeah, okay . . . Huh?

What the hell is he doing?

Dr. MacKenzie is directly to my left and there is no way I want our boss to see us playing a game at the outset of this meeting. Is Daniel trying to get me in trouble? Like making a sibling laugh while getting chewed out by Dad? Or is he trying to show me it's all a game? That he doesn't think this meeting is a big deal and neither should I? Or maybe it's a message I'm supposed to interpret in a different way: The nurses are playing a game and they've put the first X here. They're setting up the board and now it's my turn.

Being a shrink can be a real pain in the ass. I can offer up a slew of interpretations, but when the subject is me, I have to choose one all on my own, and sorting through them all is distracting me from the meeting.

People seem to be maneuvering around, trying to dodge the blame ball. Not only are the nurses giving conflicting accounts about how many patients were in the area, but now there is a discrepancy about the staffing. I'm almost positive we had fewer workers that night than they're reporting. What advantage is it for them to overstate the number of staff? At least overestimating the census makes sense to me. We were busy, we didn't catch him putting a string around his neck. But to say we were heavily staffed instead of understaffed makes us look like buffoons: We should've seen this happen if there were extra staff members tripping over one another on the unit.

The thing that makes the least sense is the nurse's triage paperwork from that night. She must have panicked. She has written not one, but three different responses in the space on the nursing triage sheet where it asks if the patient is currently suicidal. First she wrote "Vague" and then that is crossed out and it says "Denies," which is also crossed out. The third response says "I want to die."

When a patient is asked whether he is suicidal, either he says he is, or he isn't, or he's vague. Pick one! The nurse probably never got to ask him point-blank if he was suicidal. That's why she was at a loss for what to write. If she didn't get to formally interview him, why not just report that? The nurses are allowed up to two hours before they have to triage a patient, and the doctors are allowed up to six hours. Given the time frame of the events, she could've written that she hadn't asked him yet, and that would've been fine.

Luckily, Mr. Martinez hadn't been interviewed by the doctors yet, so the amount of writing I had to do in the chart was limited. I wrote one quick paragraph summing up the entire events of the night, taking the easy way out—the truth. He had been on the unit less than an hour before the suicide attempt.

Dr. MacKenzie asks me, "Dr. Holland, given what you know about the case now, in hindsight, would you have done anything different that night?"

"With hindsight I would've done everything differently, in order to prevent this suicide attempt, yes. But given what I knew prospectively, going into the case, I wouldn't have done anything differently," I answer as calmly and confidently as I can. I hope they appreciate my good grammar.

"Did you think this patient was high risk?" Dr. Henderson asks me.

"All the patients in the detainable area are high risk," I answer. I know Daniel likes my answer. We had agreed during our earlier phone call that there was nothing specific about Jesus Martinez that would have separated him out from the other patients we typically see. Nothing that was available to me at the time of his presentation, anyway.

"We see people who have just attempted suicide all the time. He wasn't particularly special in that way," I explain.

"In hindsight, everyone is a genius," Dr. MacKenzie says during the review. *Man, you aren't kidding.* I did the best I could in the moment. It was like a war zone; there was no time to mull over my options, no room for error. Now, with the luxury of time and speculation, it's all twenty-twenty vision.

The Special Review is winding down. Now that everyone who has ever treated this guy has come together, I have learned a bit more about Mr. Martinez. One new piece of information is that he had hidden a razor in his mouth on a prior visit, and a staff member saw him retrieve it from under his tongue and place it in his sock. That was one month ago, when he was admitted involuntarily to the upstairs psych unit, then transferred to the medicine floor for a work-up of a fever. He was eventually discharged home from the medical ward, instead of being transferred back to the psychiatry ward, because the psychiatrist on the consulting service said that he wouldn't benefit from an inpatient stay.

If I had known that story on Saturday night, I would've ordered a one-to-one observation for the guy as soon as he walked in the door. But I have never done that before. This was the crux of the phone conversation I had with Dr. MacKenzie prior to the one I had with Daniel.

"Wouldn't you have ordered a one-to-one on this patient as soon as he came in?" MacKenzie asked me, genuinely confused.

"Actually, we never do that." I explained. "One-to-one observations in the CPEP are very unusual. And we certainly wouldn't do that prior to an evaluation with an M.D. Don't forget, receiving a patient status-post suicide attempt is not a big deal for us." "Status-post" is a term mostly used in surgery, but I like to say it. It means "after," but it also means I went to medical school.

As the Special Review ends, I think about what I have learned. I now know that a man can want to die so badly that he will let no one stand in his way. A man such as this might make good use of a string the thickness of a hoodie tie.

CPEP will now remove the ties from zip-up sweatshirts before patients enter the detainable area. And what was once considered a high-observation area is now deemed a "blind spot." It turns out, when the nurses are at their desk filling in charts, the place where Jesus tried to end his life is invisible.

I have also learned that Mr. Martinez is still alive, still on a respirator, and will likely be transferred to a nursing home or chronic care facility. He is, for lack of a better word, a vegetable. And yet, in the ultimate rendition of closing the barn door after the horse has escaped, the nurses in the intensive care unit have ordered a one-to-one observation for him. There is a Bellevue staffer sitting by his side twenty-four hours a day to make sure he can't finish the job he very nearly completed.

No family members have come to see him as far as I know, and no one in the news media catches wind of the story, for which I am supremely thankful. I can just see the headline on the front page of the *New York Post:* SUICIDE IN THE ER! The outrage over how something like this could happen fuels my own relentless inquisition: How did I let it happen? Surely there was something that could've been done differently, that would've prevented it. I can't let it go, even after the Special Review is over.

I'm not in therapy anymore, having stopped after Molly was born. I haven't seen Mary for over a year, but I know I need to talk to someone about the suicide. I can only bend Jeremy's ear for so long before it becomes clear I need a professional to help me to process this in its entirety. I call Mary and leave a message, asking if we can have a phone session. She has a new office now, in Chelsea. It's not a convenient location for me at all, compared to her old office ten blocks from my apartment.

I remember how I convinced her I was ready to terminate, a few months after restarting, once the excitement of a new baby had died down. I felt proud of myself, getting confirmation from my therapist that I was strong enough to go on without her assistance. Now that I look back, though, I'm afraid some part of me wonders if it had more to do with her moving offices and wanting to lighten her patient load, and less to do with my readiness.

But how do we know if we're ever really done, if we're fixed? How do I know if and when I am okay? I'm married, I have a child, I have a steady job. To an outsider, I probably look pretty healthy, but am I really? I'm afraid I still haven't found that perfect balance. There has to be a middle ground between the yin and yang, the sappy and the heartless.

I need to treat the patients with compassion and dignity, but I'm afraid I'm still falling short of that goal. And now, with this suicide, I'm beating myself up for a million different reasons.

It's hard to know if I should go back into therapy or if I just need a little "booster shot," a small inoculation from Mary, a phone session to help me weather this particular storm. Whenever a patient dies in psychiatry, or in any branch of medicine, it's a big deal. But when a patient commits suicide right under your nose, practically, it's particularly unnerving, unsettling. I need help. I have to tell Mary the whole story, to unburden myself. I need her to tell me that it's all going to be okay. I feel tremendously guilty, even though there was nothing I could have done to stop it. Maybe "regret" is a better word? I relay the night's events to Mary, the phone crooked in my shoulder.

"There was nothing you could have done to stop it," Mary assures me. "You did everything you could, Julie."

Now I'm getting my money's worth.

I tell Mary how I didn't go on the offensive at the Special Review. I didn't sabotage myself. I didn't overcompensate for my guilt by making everyone else feel as bad as I did.

"Good for you," she says.

Maybe I don't need this anymore, her encouraging words. I'm spoon-feeding her everything I know she needs so she'll spoon me back what I need. Actually, I think I can probably do this for myself, finally: sidestepping the pitfalls of self-sabotage, giving myself positive feedback.

I guess I really can ride my bike without help. I just needed to be reminded of it.

Gone Daddy Gone

Daniel is leaving CPEP. He's been offered a job elsewhere at Bellevue and he's taking it. I can't imagine he's switching jobs just to get away from me, but it's certainly possible that being rid of me factored into the equation. Actually, I'm surprised he's staying at Bellevue. I thought the administration wasn't too keen on him, but I guess I was wrong. He seems pretty happy about the move, and I am dancing a jig. He is leaving and I get to stay. I can't help but feel like I've won a battle of the wills. I guess I just had to wait him out.

His gal, Michelle, is staying on, which is fine by me. They've been dating ever since that Fourth of July weekend, as far as I can tell. She's a good doctor, efficient and kind to the patients. Also, she's the new person who's organizing the moonlighter schedule. After I took my pay cut, Daniel asked her if she would take it over from me. I remember feeling unburdened as I passed along my red folder with everyone's contact information. When we sat down in her office so I could show her the ropes, I thought I'd further unburden myself. I tried to talk to her about how the whole thing played out.

"I didn't accuse Daniel of sexual harassment. I just want you to know that."

"I know," she said, staring at her computer screen. She wouldn't look at my face, and I realized we weren't going to bond over this, exactly. We would never be friends, because of all that had transpired between me and her boyfriend.

"I'm sorry you got roped into doing the scheduling. I didn't want it to go to you. I just didn't want to be the one doing it anymore," I try again, even more sincere.

"I know," she said again, still averting her gaze.

"Okay, then," I sighed heavily, giving up. "Let me show you what I have on my list."

I'm sure Michelle will eventually look for another job. She probably doesn't want to stay at CPEP under the new acting director, Maxwell. He's said some very inappropriate things about her and Daniel in the last few months, and she has absolutely no patience for him. He is quite young, probably thirty-three or thirty-four, the youngest director we've ever had. When I started at Bellevue he was a first-year resident, and not a particularly well-liked one. To fill the CPEP director vacancy, the administration went through the motions and interviewed a few people for the position, but they're not offering enough salary to entice anyone halfway decent, and Maxwell would do the job for half of what they're paying. He's just dying to be in charge.

When Daniel's secretary throws a going-away party to wish him well, she makes sure it's open bar for the first two hours. Everyone arrives on time to start drinking as much free booze as they possibly can. I sit with Julia, the social worker, and Vera and some of the other nurses. We are ordering two drinks at a time, girly drinks with straws, like daiquiris and piña coladas, tying one on in a hurry.

Daniel gets up to make a speech and everyone around me is rolling their eyes and giggling. As soon as the cake is cut, I make some excuses about having to be home early for Molly and Jeremy, and I hightail it out of there.

I make my rounds, kissing people good-bye. I am a cheek kisser or a hugger, or maybe a little bit of both. When Maxwell kisses me good-bye, I don't know if he is drunk with the power of his new position or if he is just plain trashed, but he kisses me full on the lips. I am caught off guard and wigged out. Between his saliva and one too many, I'm nauseated as I leave the restaurant, wiping my face. Julia is with me, and I complain to her about what I have just gone through.

"Eww!" she squeals like a schoolgirl.

"I know, it is eww!" I agree. We are waiting for our cabs; she's going downtown and I'm going up. I let her take the first taxi, then I climb in the back of mine. It hurls uptown, accelerating in between the stoplights and then lurching to a dead stop at the last possible minute. I feel like I'm going to hurl myself, and I have to ask the driver to chill.

"I'm not in any sort of a hurry, sir," I say as politely as I can. I lean back in the seat and remember going up this same way with Lucy back in the day, when we used to share a cab home from the faculty meetings.

I think about how different things could be now, if I had said yes instead of no. "You know I'd love you to be my assistant director, but I know you don't want it," she had said. She was right: I didn't. I was very happy working my weekend gig and had no interest in anything administrative at Bellevue. I told her Daniel was a perfectly good pick. I thought he'd be fine. But if I had taken it, Lucy and I could've rocked the house during our time together. We would've been an amazing team, with me taking care of everything at CPEP while she was sick, assuring her that it was all done to her satisfaction. And if I had said yes, I would be the director now. Me, the big boss, five days a week, running the whole show. Did I make a mistake?

It would've been the ultimate tough transition though, ascending to Lucy's throne. I know Daniel felt tortured about taking it over once Lucy was gone. When she was out sick more and more, Daniel had confided that the other division heads were talking about when he'd be the CPEP director. He hated what they intimated. He would've gladly traded Lucy's life for his promotion. It was obvious in his hesitancy. After she died, he couldn't move into her office for months. I saw all of this happening, but said nothing. Why did we never connect in our grief, in our feelings of abandonment? We could've helped each other through it, bonding over our loss instead of taking it out on each other, but neither of us extended that olive branch.

Sometimes, after I would have a fight with Daniel, I would pass by Lucy's empty office so enraged, I would give the closed door the finger. *Fuck you for leaving me here with him,* I would think. I was so angry at Lucy for leaving her post, disappearing from CPEP like an apparition. The director's office stood like a mausoleum, her name still on the door, her belongings untouched, until Sadie finally came in one weekend a few months later to clear it out. And yet even then Daniel did not move into Lucy's office.

But now, Daniel is moving on, and Maxwell will likely move into the director's office as soon as he can. Dave, Daniel's right-hand man, is leaving too. With both the director and assistant director stepping down, pickings are slim to fill the administrative positions. When MacKenzie calls me at home to get my take on whether Maxwell can do the job, I specifically mention the pie charts and graphs that Maxwell will be able to whip up for the boys upstairs. Oh, how they love their numbers. Maxwell is a computer geek extraordinaire, and he's got the social skills to go with it. I tell MacKenzie I'm okay with Maxwell in charge; he'll be fine. I know I can get away with murder with him as my boss. I've got so much seniority over him, I'm practically his mama.

Before he hangs up, MacKenzie makes a point of casually offering it to me, "Are you sure you don't want to take the position?"

"Only if I can do it working weekends," I answer breezily. It's become my stock answer every time someone asks me if I want the director's job. I know it isn't a realistic option and it's fine with me. I've been happy doing my two shifts a week and I have no desire for more. When I'm there, I'm in charge, and that's enough for me.

Maxwell will be my fourth director in only eight years at CPEP. Meet the new boss, same as the old boss. But I am sorry Daniel and I were never able to resolve our differences. We just couldn't make it work with Lucy gone. We should have forged a friendship in her honor, but the time for that has passed. I'm staying. He's going. And here comes my new supervisor. Maxwell will be a cinch compared to Daniel, and I won't be reminded of Lucy's absence quite so acutely.

All the Rage

Every Friday, I take the 6 train downtown to see my private patients. I am in my Greenwich Village office with a thirtysomething working gal. My practice is packed with them: Single and dating but not finding "the one," they get more anxious and depressed as they round the corner to forty. Manhattan is full of pharmacies distributing oral contraceptives and antidepressants with my name on the bottle.

We are twenty minutes into our half-hour session; she has her prescriptions and we're making small talk before I prepare her bill. Her cell phone rings and I motion for her to take it. It's fine with me, I have paperwork to do.

"Hello?" she asks, tentatively. "No, I can't talk. I'm with my psychopharmacologist," she sings, the seven-syllable word trilling from her mouth. There is no secrecy or hesitation in her voice, but rather a sense of entitlement, of gloating: *I have one, don't you have one too?*

I have become the equivalent of a Prada handbag.

A psychopharm is not a therapist, but rather someone who specializes in psychiatric medications. There is no lying down on my couch and talking about your traumatic childhood or what you dreamed last night. I ask you about specific symptoms, and then fix up just the right cocktail to get you back on your feet. One of the reasons I believe so strongly in psychopharmacology is that it works. And it is fast. Good psychotherapy takes years: Personal growth comes slowly; there is no straight trajectory, and it's not always obvious whether the therapy is working or not. Antidepressants and mood stabilizers help to eradicate many symptoms of psychiatric syndromes. People feel better and their lives become less chaotic when a good combination of medications are chosen and adhered to.

"Don't ask the barber if you need a haircut."

This quote was on the wall at Mount Sinai, next to the X-ray light boxes. If asked for an opinion, the radiologist would often recommend another study to follow up the first. A barber makes his money cutting hair. Could you use a trim? Sure! If you have a condition that can be managed medically or surgically, what kind of advice do you think the surgeon will give you?

People who come to me are stressed-out and anxious or depressed. They have concerns about their sleep, their mood, their level of energy and motivation. These things can be ameliorated with medication, and I tell them so. Every once in a while I will still get a patient who is un-sure if he should take medication or not. I take a thorough history and an inventory of family diagnoses of mood disorders. I ask for details about any chemical manipulations that have already been experienced (coffee, cigarettes, pot, psychedelic mushrooms, Ecstasy, various pre-scription medications borrowed from friends) to help me get a sense of what will feel most comfortable.

People have this idea that they have a "chemical imbalance." That may well be true, but there is no simple test to determine exactly where your balance may be off. I learn about a patient's symptoms, gene pool, self-medication preferences, and then I synthesize that into a best guess—a medication to start with.

Sometimes I'll compare what I do to the job of an optometrist who asks, "Better like this? Better like that?" as he takes two minutes to pick out the perfect lens. I do the same thing, but sometimes it takes months as I try different combinations of medications.

I try to assure my patients, "I have a good feel for this, for whatever reason. My intuition helps out, and I usually get it right on the first try. Sometimes we'll have to try a second medication, or a combination of two medicines, but I'll aim for happy and relaxed, with a minimum of side effects. It could happen in a few weeks, or a few months, but we'll get you back to your old self again."

A patient who believes in me will believe in my ability to heal. That translates into faith in whatever I prescribe, and when this happens, we're more than halfway there. The placebo effect looms large in all of medicine, but it probably matters most in psychiatry. When I pick a medication, I really try to sell it. It helps that I mostly prescribe the meds I really like, the ones that I've seen work like magic.

Typically, a few months down the road, the next talk we have occurs when the patient is feeling better. "How long can I take this for?" The unspoken belief: It's not okay to take these pills forever. It's not normal to feel this good. There must be a catch.

It takes some getting used to, the idea that a little pill, swallowed daily, can provide such substantial relief. Some people adjust to this new fact of life, and others fight it. I encourage my patients to stay on their medications for at least six months, to get comfortable with being comfortable. Many people feel better than they've ever felt, and that feels awkward. Whether it's okay to stay medicated or not is a thorny issue. Most people will feel better on meds than off, but there are some instances where prescriptions should provide only short-term relief. I usually offer two different analogies, and let the patients pick the most appropriate one.

"Say you have unequal-length legs. If I give you a shoe with a higher heel, you can walk normally, barely noticing the discrepancy. But when you remove the shoe, you'll have trouble walking again. If you have a predisposition toward anxiety or depression, medications will relieve your symptoms, but they won't change your natural tendency. If we stop the medicines, you'll most likely go back to feeling the way you did before."

The contrasting analogy I like to use is the "pillow under the butt" scenario: "Say you're going down a bumpy road in an old jalopy. You feel every rock; you're practically thrown from the car. The medicine is like a cushion for your seat. You won't get so derailed by the stressors in your life. Maybe over time your path will become smoother, or maybe through psychotherapy your jalopy will turn into a luxury car with better shock absorbers. Then you won't need the pillow anymore."

I have seen over time that the shoe analogy is more apt. My patients stay with me for years, trying various combinations of medications to defend them from their own misfiring chemistry, exacerbated by the pressures of city living. Their paths rarely become smoother, and even

if the psychotherapy is terribly successful, they still find that they feel
better when they have that extra cushion that medication provides.

So what do we talk about once they're stable on their regimens and
we aren't making many changes? As a psychopharmacologist, I don't officially do psychotherapy per se, but there are always important things
to talk about even when the medications don't need to be adjusted. I
establish what could be called a "holding environment," in which to
care for my patients. Basically, I try to preach what I practice. I share
with my patients what I've figured out so far. I urge them to exercise;
consistent cardio does wonders for depression and anxiety, I tell them.
I remind them to breathe deeply when they're tense. "Never underesti-
mate the power of oxygen," I say.

I focus on harm reduction, as opposed to abstinence. People are going to use substances to alter their consciousness—that is simply a fact
of life. And life in the Big Apple is fast-paced and overwhelming. My
patients work hard, long hours. With cell phones and BlackBerrys, the
scarcity of downtime is a common theme. They use food, alcohol, and
other drugs to help them relax. Adding shame to their burden is coun-
terproductive. I'm not judgmental when they admit their vices to me,
but I will remind them about running and yoga, the *Power of Now,* and
"just doing nothing" as healthier alternatives. I encourage integration
of relaxation and contentment into their jam-packed schedules, and I
remind them to have fun, lighten up, and stay in the moment.

Our culture, more than most others, has a hard time incorporating
pleasure into the daily routine. Indulging ourselves makes us nervous.
There is an element of guilt that accompanies fulfilling our own needs,
so we binge secretly, quickly. We women, especially, seem uncomfortable nourishing ourselves, and self-neglect is common. We give to others readily, but to ourselves rarely.

Mostly, I'm starting to realize that psychiatry is primarily projected
self-care. I give my patients what I can't seem to fully give myself: atten-
tive nurturing, compassion, gentle understanding. I'm still struggling
with many of the basic issues that my patients are, though it's easier for
me and for them to think that I have it all down pat. I don't let on that I
am a wounded healer, as fragile and fallible as anyone else.

The ultimate goal of psychotherapy is self-love and self-acceptance.
It is elusive, but I try to model the desired behavior. My own psychotherapist, Mary, taught me to be loving and gentle with myself, mostly

by setting an example for me to emulate. She helped me tame my own self-destruction, and now I am carrying her torch, helping others to trade in their masochism in favor of self-preservation. If I can show my patients enough love and acceptance, maybe they can join me in feeling good about themselves. If they think I'm happy and relaxed, it might make it easier for them to try it.

Making healthy choices is an awkward behavior that takes years to master. Not beating yourself up when you slow down is a good first step. Most of my patients are unmercifully hard on themselves. Happy and relaxed feels unearned and undeserved, foreign and frightening. What is more comfortable and familiar is shame, humiliation, and guilt. These are ingrained by family and society. We binge and purge on cycles of indulgence and regret. Gratify yourself, punish yourself.

We dance on the borderline, the shifting boundary of grandiosity and inadequacy. After hubris comes humiliation, when the idealized version of ourselves doesn't jibe with reality, and those internalized, derisive voices sure can kick us when we're down. This sets off a rebellious anger that is directed nowhere but inward. Too often, there is no effective defense from the bullying. It simply triggers more self-destructive behavior.

We don't see what's clean; we only see what's dirty, what is contemptible in the eyes of our inner critic. We can focus on improvements yet to be made, yes, but we should also give ourselves credit for our achievements. There is a lot to be said for gratitude, and for accentuating the positive. I remind my patients to appreciate all they have and all they've accomplished, to embrace their largesse and abundance instead of focusing on what they fear is missing or imperfect.

My private practice patients are aware of my Bellevue patients. Sometimes I will hear an embarrassing confession, followed by, "Does that sound crazy?"

I'm able to say, "You want crazy? Let me tell you a little story," before launching into a Bellevue tale to help put things in perspective. I think it helps them to know that I see people who are substantially sicker than they are.

Bellevue is the perfect yang to my Greenwich Village office yin. At CPEP, I am faced with sequential catastrophes as I put out fires. I triage red, yellow, or green and move on to the next disaster. In my office, it's more about preventative care, like seeing the dentist regularly and being reminded to brush and floss. Waiting until symptoms and problems have reached epic proportions is hardly the optimal time for intervention. At Bellevue, the patients are nearly toothless, to extend the metaphor. I can only do so much in a twenty-minute CPEP interview, and the dysfunctionality of "the system" itself gets in my way. The patients bounce from hospital to shelter to jail to hospital.

In my office, without my cowboy chaps, I am softer, less protected, and more connected. I can inch forward, opening myself up, and have more hope that I can make a difference. And I don't get burnt out. On the contrary, I get back as much as I give.

At CPEP, I can't tolerate getting close because the stories are just too intense. The hardships that my patients endure are like an abyss, threatening to engulf me. But I do need to be touching people's lives more. I am learning that now. I used to think I could never do full-time private practice without CPEP to balance it out. I thought I would get bored.

Now I'm not so sure.

Whatever Gets You Through the Night

I walk into the CPEP to start yet another shift. It is the fall of 2003, my eighth year. The waiting area looks like a precinct: An assortment of irritated, swearing, drunken arrestees are flanked by two uniformed cops each.

The resident has other patients to see and the police cases are rarely educational. All of these guys are mine as far as I'm concerned. This could take most of my night.

When I started in 1996, we were doing pre-arraignment evaluations for Manhattan and the Bronx only. Now we've opened up our catchment area to all five boroughs. Anyone arrested in New York City who seems a little off, or happens to be taking any psychotropic medication, has to pass though our doors. These days, nearly half of all the patients coming through CPEP are under arrest. I'm plenty interested in forensics, but there's just so much cops and robbers a gal can take.

And then there's the paperwork. Recently, in the name of efficiency, the forms we fill out on each patient have changed. But, like any form made by committee, it's got even more boxes to check off than before, and it is insufferably long. I'm spending more time writing than I am interviewing, by far. Anyway, enough bellyaching. I gotta get to work.

The loudest patients are always my number one priority. A very large transgender male to female patient, her eyebrows shaped and nails painted, has been brought in screaming and crying. Three pre-arraignments? Make that four.

"Are you ready for this one, Doc?" the cop asks me.

"I was born ready, Sarge," I volley back. (I like to talk like I'm on television whenever I can.)

"This guy, this lady, whatever. He threw a container of piss at a bus driver!"

I stare at the cop, not sure I heard him right. "Urine?" I ask. "In a container?"

The patient is crying dramatically, "I'm sorry! I'm sorry! Don't hurt me! Don't hurt me!"

"Ma'am," I begin softly. "Miss? Can you tell me what happened?" It is always most polite to address transgender patients in their preferred gender. Clearly this man has gone through a lot of trouble to be appreciated as a woman. It is an easy way for me to convey to him that I get it, I respect his mission.

"Don't hurt me! Please, don't hurt me!"

"I'm not going to hurt you. No one here is going to hurt you. We just want you to calm down so we can help you. Can you answer some questions for us?"

"I'm sorry! I'm sorry!"

"Do you know where you are? Can you tell me your name?"

"I'm sorry! Don't hurt me! I'm sorry!"

Is she psychotic? The cop's story sounds like she could have been. Or, it could have been more drama than insanity. The way she's acting now, she seems like she's stuck inside some sort of dramatic episode, just crying and crying. Maybe something that's happening now is resonating with a past traumatic event? She's not obviously hallucinating or paranoid, but she is unable to focus on anything but her misery and so can't attend to any other stimuli. In that way, you could say that she is broken from reality, and in effect psychotic.

Nancy is the head nurse on with me tonight. She stands before me with her hands on her wide hips, all business. "What you wanna do with this one, Julie?"

"Can we give her Ativan four IM?" I ask, undecided. I'm open to suggestions, as usual, which is why I don't state it as a command. Nancy takes my request as if it is an order, stated more definitively, which is how we prefer to play it most nights. If she has a problem with my medication order, she won't shy away from letting me know, though it probably won't be spoken. Usually, we do a lot of talking in CPEP with our eyebrows, not our mouths.

The patient lets Nancy give her the injection, amazingly. "Good thing she didn't fight it, cause that is one humongous she-male!" I exclaim, relieved, when we are on the other side of the glass.

After the Ativan starts to kick in, the patient quiets down, looking around the nondetainable area like a little kid, lost in Wonderland. I assign her to the resident after all, who goes out to get the full story.

"So, what's her deal?" I ask, putting my feet up on the desk, waiting for the resident to present the case to me.

"Okay, so she was on this bus, right? A ninety-minute bus ride from Rockland down to the city."

"State hospital Rockland?" I ask, my eyebrows at attention.

"Yeah, but she says she doesn't go there for treatment. I asked."

"Good thinking, asking."

"So, she's on this long bus ride and she needs to go to the bathroom. But there is no bathroom on the bus, so she asks the bus driver to let her off somewhere, but he won't. So she went to the back of the bus and urinated into some sort of plastic bottle and then threw it at him 'cause she was mad at him for not stopping."

"Okay, well, our job is just to make sure she's not psychotic, suicidal, or homicidal. So far she's just assaultive and showing poor judgment, poor impulse control, et cetera."

"Right. But now, her main concern is that the police are going to abuse her, and she's afraid of the other prisoners doing the same. The cops are going to take her to central booking, right?"

"I guess so. But they must have a separate area for the transgender prisoners. I know they do at Rikers." I throw my feet down, and get up from my chair. "Let's go ask the cops."

I am amazed at how calm the patient is now. "You see this? This is great!" I open my arms wide toward the becalmed Babe in Toyland. I am trying to teach the resident something. "Ativan four is my favorite first-line med for sedating a triage. The more I use it, the more I like it better than Haldol five and Ativan two. Look at how calm she is! You give five and two, you incapacitate the patient and it makes further interviews and interactions impossible for at least eight hours. I thought for sure we'd have to eat this admission because the cops wouldn't be able to deal with the screaming and the drama. And I was afraid it'd take a mess of meds to get her quiet, and then she'd sleep for days. The Ativan four really allows her to calm down and get herself together, but not turn her into a zombie. So now, she can leave!" I say this last part excitedly as we are getting closer to the patient's stretcher.

"Ma'am? Are you almost ready to go?" I ask her in a quieter voice, turning on the concerned, therapeutic, caring charm.

"It's not safe," she tells us in a stage whisper. "They don't understand me."

"Sweetheart, I promise you. You are not the first transgender prisoner in NYPD's history."

We assure her that the police will be considerate and she has nothing to fear. Soon, she calms down enough to leave.

Nancy is pleasantly surprised. It is a magical transformation, and we are both singing the praises of Ativan four, the wonder drug that works wonders.

The second patient is a guy who was initially brought to the medical ER after he was arrested for shoplifting. He told the cops he had a hernia, but the AES was unimpressed with his bulge, deeming it non-emergent, so they sent him to the corrections holding area to wait for transport to arraignment. While in the blue room, the patient somehow attempted to hang himself using his leg irons. This is a new one on me. He must be awfully flexible and ingenious. The police bring him to CPEP where he is yelling and spitting to beat the band. He is mostly calling the police officers names, screaming how they're all faggots and they can suck his dick. Once he is tied down and sedated, they begin to search him, emptying his pockets, taking off his shoes. He needs to be searched before he enters the detainable area, and I am nearly positive we'll have to admit him.

The cops find two bottles of nitroglycerin sublingual tablets in his pockets, and one bottle of heparin in his shoe. Evidently, he has stolen these from the medical ER. The nitro is a medication that dilates the heart's blood vessels, meant to be given to a person in the midst of acute chest pain. The heparin is an intravenous medication used to prevent blood clots from forming. If he had swallowed even one bottle of the tablets, it could have been a medical emergency, but I'm not sure he knows the value of what he has filched, and I'm even less sure he had any intention of actually hurting himself. He may have thought he could sell them on the street.

I can't get much out of him during the interview, though he's much calmer with me than he was with the police, and there is no talk of fellatio. He is a flamboyantly gay Filipino male who is quick to report his bipolar diagnosis. He seems entirely believable to me, as he tells me his psychiatrist's name and number, which he chants rhythmically like a Sousa march. This is the verse: name and number, name and number. When he gets to the chorus, he switches to his lawyer's name and number. He repeats them both so often and so distinctly that I do not need to write them down. I have the song in my head for the rest of my shift.

I leave a message with the psychiatrist who calls me back fairly quickly. This sort of thing happens a lot, it sounds like. We have a great conversation, bonding over our love of our jobs, and he fills me in on the patient's most recent medication regimen. He's been switching around some of his meds, and we chat until we agree on a pharmacological plan of action. I fill out the admissions paperwork, meticulously ordering all the meds per our discussion, hoping the up-wards docs continue them as written.

My third prisoner is making his Christmas wish list a little early. It is only mid-September, but he is unabashedly asking for methadone, Clonidine, and Klonipin. Three different sedatives, one of which is a potent opioid narcotic, similar in its effects to heroin. He has seen me give Ativan 4 IM to prisoner number one, and he wants to know why he hasn't been seen and medicated yet.

"What do I have to do to get some Ativan around here? Do I gotta bust up this joint?" he shouts.

His police escorts stand idly by, surveying the scene but opting not to intervene. I stand in front of the prisoner and say, "If this guy acts up, give him twenty-five of Thorazine IM." I say this to the resident while staring at the patient.

The prisoner quiets down. This tells me plenty. He knows his drugs. He knows Thorazine will make him feel absolutely horrid. He knows I mean business, and if he's a good little boy, maybe he'll get a treat. I may feel charitable and give him one of the sedatives on his wish list. But if he's bad, he'll get the charcoal in his stocking.

The fourth prisoner is an ornery man, rude and irritable. He has tattoos of letters on his fingers and on his neck. The fingers are a tip-off that he's been in jail, and the neck is typically a warning sign that I'm dealing with a sociopath. He's giving the police a hard time, but when he gets alone in an interview room with the medical student, he is sweet as pie, subservient, calling her Miss and Ma'am interchangeably. He won't tell her what he is arrested for, or what he has been in prison for in the past, but he does tell her that he takes Prozac 100 mg and Ativan 50 mg. He says "BID," which stands for twice a day, so he has done his homework, except that these are outrageously high doses, so even though he's calm and seemingly cooperative, he's lying through his teeth.

He also reports that he gets 130 mg of methadone a day and says he is in withdrawal, because he hasn't had any in several days. This is a high dose, but not an uncommon one. However, his pupils aren't dilated and he doesn't have any goose bumps on his skin. These are two physical manifestations of opiate withdrawal that are difficult to manufacture, so it's an easy way for me to check his story.

He denies being suicidal, homicidal, or psychotic, so I get the paperwork together to send him out with the police.

I walk out into the nondetainable area to talk to the police officer on the case. The cop is a jaded, older guy who tells me he is close to retirement. I always think of Danny Glover in *Lethal Weapon* when I hear a cop say he's nearly retiring. Glover's character ends up getting roped into a dangerous and complicated case just days before he can leave the police force in one piece, which makes me nervous during the whole movie.

This officer tells me he's taking a course to become a respiratory therapist. He has a house in upstate New York and is hoping to get a job in a hospital near there. He mentions he has PTSD and asthma from 9/11, so I guess he must've been down there and seen some horrible things. He is sharing an awful lot with me, more than the average officer, and it finally occurs to me why. He is trying to butter me up because he wants the guy sedated. Tonight, everyone is trying to get on my good side to get the good drugs.

The prisoner has been giving him a hard time, and he is in no mood. The cop is at the end of his rope, nearing the end of his time in the force, and he is running out of steam. He also tells me what his prisoner would not, which is that the charge is rape, and he's been imprisoned in the past for the same.

"If you're going to release him to me, can you please medicate the hell out of him?" the cop finally asks me.

I reply as I often do, "Happy and compliant or dead weight?"

The cop answers wearily, but without skipping a beat, "If this guy isn't dead weight, I'm afraid I'm gonna have to kill him."

"Sir?" I ask, just to make sure I heard him right. He isn't saying it like he's kidding; he's saying it like he's exhausted, and it's the path of least resistance.

"Dead weight, dead prisoner, what's the difference? The guy's a rapist," the cop moans.

Wow. Did I say jaded? It's clearly time for this officer to begin his new career as a respiratory therapist upstate, and head out to pasture. Stick a fork in him; he's done.

"Right-O," I say cheerfully. "I'll see what I can do for you, sir." Best to just remain polite and let it go. This cop is not my patient.

I unlock the door to leave the waiting room and I am hit with a blast of noise in the detainable area. The arrested rapist is now all over me for his methadone, no more mister nice guy. He's gone from catching flies with honey to spewing vinegar in my face.

"The hospital limits us to how much methadone we can administer," I explain. I don't specify the amount, because I know he'll blow his top if he hears it's only twenty milligrams.

"Call my methadone clinic and they'll tell you the dose!" he screams at me, his face contorting and reddening.

"Sir, it's eleven o'clock at night on a Sunday. There's no one at your clinic right now."

"Someone is there. Someone is always there," he insists.

I go inside to talk to Nancy. "The cop wants dead weight, the prisoner wants methadone. Looks like we should probably just take advantage of the situation." We agree to do something that everyone knows damn well is completely against the rules. I have never done it before or since: I tell the patient we're going to give him an injection of methadone, and we give him Thorazine.

I tell the medical student, "This is the first time in my seven years at Bellevue that I am ever doing this. It's medically unethical what we are doing, do you understand? You never lie to a patient about what medicine they are getting; it's against all the rules. Actually, I'm pretty sure it's against the law. But sometimes down here, the end justifies the means. This way, he calms down, the cop is happy, they both leave and we go on with our night."

The medical student nods earnestly. She understands; she doesn't see any problem with what we are doing. She'll make a good ER doc some-day, and I tell her so. I, on the other hand, am starting to see myself in a new light, beginning to feel that two-shades-beyond-golden-brown, burnt-out feeling creeping up on me. I'm not quite "crispy" yet, but I'm getting there.

Your Mother Should Know

Flashback: Saturday afternoon, September 11, 1999. After I go running in the park and shower, Jeremy and I have sex before I leave for work.

As I walk down the back hallway toward my office, I notice a sharp, twisting pain in my right lower quadrant: I can actually feel myself ovulate. I get very excited, convinced the timing has been perfect and Jeremy and I have successfully conceived our first child. It is our first time trying; we have been married for four months.

I have a few minutes before my shift starts to go to the coffee shop to get something for dinner. In the line, I run into my friend Gideon, a social worker at CPEP. I decide to let him in on my secret, unable to contain myself, as usual.

"Guess what?" I ask him.

"What?" he responds, excitedly. Gideon can get enthused about anything. He's the perfect person to tell, because he'll mirror back all my elation and then some.

"I'm pregnant, I think. And you are the very first to know."

"Oh my God! That is so amazing! How far along are you?" he asks.

"What time is it?" I answer.

Three weeks later, I pee on a stick and the plus sign appears. We have gone from newlyweds in May to expectant parents in September in the blink of an eye, and we are almost a teensy bit disappointed that we didn't get to spend a few more months trying.

Be careful what you wish for.

Conceiving our second child is a completely different ball game. I am four years older, now thirty-eight, and we are at it for well over a year. I complain constantly about what a pain in the ass it is. ("I know, I know. Then we're doing it wrong!" I joke with the coffee shop guy.) In all seriousness, I am growing a bit tired of doing it with Jeremy. Baby-making is not sexy. It is like a job you have to show up for, even though you want to sleep in. All the romance has gone out of it; we are slaves to my cycle, my erratic temperature chart, the consistency of my cervical mucus. I take the thermometer to Bellevue on the weekends and lie down impatiently in my office on Sunday and Monday mornings, waiting to get my basal temperature readings before I get out of bed to prepare for sign-out.

We have sex every other night during my fertile week, whether we want to or not. *You again!* I think to myself as we try to gear up to get off yet again. *Jeez, can I please get someone new over here?*

We try month after month, to no avail.

There is one day up at the house when we stick Molly in front of the television to watch *Snow White* as we run upstairs to our bedroom. I try to get "Whistle While You Work" out of my head to better get in the mood. We are giggling as we hear her video playing downstairs, and I have a funny feeling I'm not going to feel the same way about those dwarves in the future.

After fifteen months of unsuccessful attempts, I finally give in and take Clomid, a medicine that causes more eggs to be released during ovulation. I am deathly afraid of twins, but what I get instead is a few days of industrial-strength premenstrual moodiness.

On a Monday night up at the house, I insist to Jeremy that tonight's the night. I'm so tired, having worked two overnights with no sleep in between due to having one child already. The last thing I want to do is get it on, really, but it's nonnegotiable. I have taken the Clomid and the timing is perfect. It's now or never.

When we are done, I have a powerful sense that it has worked—call it women's intuition, maternal instinct, or magical thinking. Jeremy gets up to go to the bathroom, and I say something softly to the new being cooking in my pelvis. "Stay with us, little man. We want you here with us. You're in the right place. Stay."

The Clomid does work, thankfully, and soon after, my uterus acts like a balloon that's already been blown up once before. There is no resistance, and I start to show immediately. Nancy tells me one day, "Julie, when you was pregnant with Molly, your butt got really wide. But this time, you gettin' a bubble butt. It's going straight out. That's why we think you having a boy this time."

"We?" I ask, bracing myself for what I know is coming.

"Yeah. The nurses."

"So, you all stand around here and discuss the dimensions of my ass?"

"Only when you're pregnant!" She grins.

I have turned into the doctor with a three-year-old at home and another one on the way. "Going another round, eh?" is a popular question around the hospital. There's no denying it now, no pretending I'm hip anymore. I've joined the parenthood club, hook, line, and sinker. At Bellevue, the staff who have kids seem to know everyone else; the status of our children is the currency we use to exchange pleasantries. I discuss toilet training with the hospital police officers, sleep strategies with the radiology technician, and the fertility tricks I've learned with the man behind the counter at the coffee shop. It is a level of intimacy atypical for colleagues, but the folks at Bellevue feel like family. Actually, I see them more often than any of my relatives.

There is one hospital police officer, Pablo, who has a child Molly's age. He never fails to ask me how Molly's doing, and he loves to show me the latest photo of his daughter. He's split up with his wife recently, and I know it must kill him to have limited contact with his girl. I see the way his sunny face clouds over when I ask him about it.

I come to work one Saturday to learn that Pablo's daughter has been struck by a van in a hit-and-run accident. She is transferred to Bellevue from another hospital, but it doesn't look good. She's on life support, and from what I can gather from the other officers, she may be brain-dead. The entire ground floor of the hospital, where the HP headquarters and most of the security checkpoints are located, is eerily quiet.

Pablo is friendly and well-liked, and the staff speak in private whispers, gathering in twos and threes in the corners to discuss the latest on the girl's medical condition. I keep an eye out for him so that I may express my sympathies, to see if there's anything I can do, but I don't see him around.

Later in the weekend, I find out that she has in fact died.

When I do finally see Pablo, I am too upset to speak to him. The lump in my throat forbids it. Tears sting my eyes at the sight of him, the thought of his anguish. I don't know how it is that he can pull himself together to be back at the job so soon, but then I realize he's only come in to do some paperwork so he can take a leave of absence. He is dressed in a suit and tie, as opposed to his usual blue HP uniform, and he seems to have aged a decade since I saw him last. I can't even imagine the pain he must be feeling. I turn away, feigning absorption in some other task, feeling ashamed at not being man enough to approach him.

It is the ultimate undoing, the pain of losing a child. More often than not, it does irreparable damage. I have seen countless patients who pinpoint their psychiatric decline to the date of their son or daughter's death. Marriages crumble, and individuals disintegrate.

I should go to him. I should hug him, tell him the same thing everyone else is telling him, "If there's anything I can do . . ." But I do nothing. I say nothing. There are multiple opportunities for me to pay my respects and acknowledge his situation, but I escape them all as my avoidance snowballs over time. Somehow, I cannot align my motherhood—our shared parenthood—with my steely Bellevue doctor persona; I cannot tolerate the bleed-through between my two compartmentalized existences.

I remember the closest I ever got to losing Molly, the twenty-seconds-of-terror vortex that sucked all other reality out of existence. She was nine months old and eating a yogurt-covered pretzel. She liked to suck the vanilla coating off the pretzels, but she didn't like to eat the pretzels themselves, so I would finish up the job from there.

I left her sitting in the middle of the living room floor as I was putting away the laundry in the bedroom. And then I realized it was very quiet, and quite still. Too still. I popped my head into the living room and checked on Molly. She was sitting on the floor as before, but she was red in the face. A high-pitched whistle, very faint, was coming from somewhere in the living room.

It was coming from her.

She was choking on the pretzel, moving just enough air to create this reedy sound, looking up at me with wide-open eyes.

I picked her up and put her over my knee with my foot on the couch. I hit her back hard, angling her head down. Whap! Whap! Whap!

Nothing.

Oh my God, oh my God. She's choking to death. She's not moving any air.
The squeal was dying out. Her face was getting more dusky.
Is she going to die? I can't get the pretzel out!
What do I do? You're not supposed to Heimlich a little baby. What else can I do? I have to do something.

I spun her around and put my fist in her stomach, lifting her up against it. I not only Heimliched her, I did it with all her weight against my fist.

Pop.

The pretzel sailed across the couch.

She began to wail.

I started to breathe again.

I held her tight, squeezing her to me, trying to calm myself down so I could calm her down.

No more pretzels.

Before Molly was born, as my wedding date neared, Mary had asked me how I would feel if Jeremy died. I don't remember what brought this up, but I do remember answering that of course I would be heartbroken, but that eventually I would pick up the pieces and get on with my life, and down the road I would probably even fall in love again. She may have been surprised by the coldness of my answer, but I was getting used to my usual defense against any kind of loss or pain.

But now, when I think about how I would handle Molly's death, I'm not so sure I could go on. It feels more accurate to think that if she died, I would have to die as well. I couldn't tolerate the pain.

How will Pablo handle his pain? And what can I possibly say or do for him that would offer him any real comfort? To murmur the same lines as everyone else—"My heart goes out to you. I am so sorry for your loss."—what does that accomplish?

As my years go by at Bellevue, and I clock in more time, the stakes keep getting higher. The threat of loss looms larger now that I have people depending on me. It's not just my survival, which never was that big a priority. I notice with my second pregnancy that I am thinking more in terms of my family, and how to keep it intact. I must stay healthy and safe so I can take care of them. I begin to feel more at risk, the way I did after I was punched. It's the little things now, not just intimidating patients: for instance, the shampoo we use to kill lice. It's toxic to a fetus, and pregnant women can't be exposed to it. With new regard, I look at the bottles lying around the nurses' station and shudder as I put on a pair of gloves and move them to the locked area where we store medications.

Once again, as I start to show with my second pregnancy, the nurses won't let me go out into the patient area unless it is absolutely necessary. They treat me like a delicate, though bloated, hothouse flower, and I enjoy the pampering that comes with my gestation. I start spending more time in the nurses' area doing paperwork, and less time going out to meet the patients in the triage area. I especially don't go onto the unit if a patient is escalating and will likely require restraints, the way I would've in the past.

It gets boring, having less patient contact, but it also makes me feel cared for, knowing that the nurses are watching out for me, protecting me and my family as if I were a part of their family. And they're right; a pregnant doctor does need extra protection.

A few years ago, when I was pregnant with Molly, a new television show called *Wonderland* came on the air. The creator and writers had befriended the Bellevue staff, and had observed how CPEP and the wards were run. In one episode, the female CPEP attending, who also happened to be pregnant, got stabbed in the belly with a hypodermic needle, injuring her fetus. She was doing a consult on a patient in the medical ER. The morning after that show aired, Daniel made a joke about it at rounds, saying how I, the pregnant psychiatrist, could go to the AES to do consults if any got called in. We all laughed, myself included, though I remember thinking he was such an asshole to say that. But I also remember feeling nervous. What if some nut job saw the show and it gave him an idea?

Then there was the nagging memory of the pregnant pathologist who was strangled at Bellevue before I began working there. Six months along and choked to death. I thought of her often while I walked the empty corridors late at night during both my pregnancies.

Besides stabbings and stranglings, there are also infections to worry about. When Molly was about a year old, there were two weekends when CPEP was under quarantine. Some patients had come down with Norovirus, a virulent GI virus that had recently wreaked havoc on a cruise ship. The good news was that CPEP was shut down. We couldn't admit any more patients into the area, so EMS diversion was a hard-and-fast rule, not a courtesy; I could actually turn ambulances away. After two weekends, the census got down to zero. Someone took pictures of the empty hallways and stretchers, labeling the Polaroids stuck to the wall "The Perfect CPEP." I had spent the bulk of my shifts watching DVDs and eating microwave popcorn.

Coming in for work that first night, it was exciting to see the doctors and nurses wearing yellow paper gowns and masks. But then, I realized there was a chance I could carry home the virus, spreading it to my husband and daughter. Norovirus causes so much vomiting and diarrhea that children can die from dehydration. When I got home the next morning, I stood at the doorway, afraid to walk into our apartment, afraid to hug them hello. When Jeremy asked me what was the matter, I wanted him to hold me and comfort me, but I felt contaminated and contagious.

How am I going to keep working at a job that's potentially life-threatening not just to myself, but to my children? I can't keep placing us all in harm's way.

But the next Saturday night, and the ones after that, I drive down to Bellevue, gearing up for another round.

Leaving the Note

I have a manila folder full of suicide notes.

For a while at Bellevue, if I came across one at my job, I would Xerox it and add it to my file. Eventually, I stopped doing this. It became overstuffed and sadly redundant and meaningless. There are few things as demoralizing as a stack of suicide notes—all that hopelessness, so much sorrow and regret concentrated in one place. It's unnatural.

Some of the notes are apologetic:

"Tell Ilana I'm sorry."

"I know I'm hurting you by what I'm about to do, but I see no other way out of this."

"I am so sad and so sorry. Please forgive me."

But there are plenty of notes full of anger, not apologies.

One note, addressed to an ex-boyfriend, says succinctly, "This is all your fault."

At least the notes make it easy for me to make a decision about how to handle the case. They are tangible proof that a patient wants to die, which allows me to fill out the paperwork for the admission. The problem is, not everyone leaves a note, and even if they've written one, it doesn't always signify seriousness or intention. Plenty of completed suicides leave no note. And plenty of staged suicidal gestures are accompanied by long letters.

Sometimes a patient will make a veiled or outright threat of suicide on the phone. The person on the other end of the call, not knowing what else to do, dials 911. Then I get a new angry patient showing up in CPEP, dragged out of his home by EMS, forced against his will to undergo a psychiatric evaluation.

One of the rules of thumb that I've developed over the years is to base my treatment plan not on what someone says, but on what he does. People threaten suicide for all sorts of dramatic reasons. I try not to take away their civil liberties and force them into a Bellevue stay unless I have proof of actual harmful intent. Dramatic phone calls don't count. I've had countless situations where the ex-boyfriend calls 911 after the girl he dumped threatens to kill herself. She was hoping he'd come rescue her, but what she gets instead are a couple of ambulance drivers escorting her to a night with me. Now she has to convince me that she has things to live for. Lucky for her, I'm not hard to convince. I let most people leave the CPEP as soon as we've had a quick chat, once I get the feeling that they have "future thinking." I write up a T & R, documenting that a patient has no suicidal intent, is not hopeless, and has future plans and future thinking. These are key components in the decision to release a patient.

It's tough to decide who's really serious about suicide, whom to detain. Anyone who's recently made an attempt is an automatic keeper; that's easy. Talking about it is one thing—threatening, writing notes, those are things that will make me consider an admission—but if they went through with any sort of dangerous activity, they're in, end of story.

It is standard practice when evaluating a recent suicide attempt to do a "walk-through." I ask the patient to take me through that whole day, step by step, to get a sense of how much thought and planning went into the attempt, if any. What were the thoughts and hopes while carrying it out? Many attempts are impulsive and barely thought out. Other times, people will admit that they were hoping to be thwarted, that a loved one would finally understand just how desperate things had become.

Another situation that comes up every once in a while is "suicide by cop." Patients, usually psychotic or high on cocaine or both, will try to get the police to kill them with their guns. Sometimes they will do this by trying to provoke aggression. Other times, they'll reach for the cop's gun, trying to get it out of the holster, which is trickier than it looks—I've tried it (with permission, of course).

Obviously, patients who successfully commit suicide don't cross my path. They go to the medical ER to be resuscitated, or they go to the morgue. The patients that I do see are the failed suicide attempts. The note has been found in time, or the patient is discovered in the bathroom with a noose around his neck, or in the tub with his wrists cut and bleeding.

These are the most pathetic things that I deal with, bar none—the botched suicides. It's not that easy to successfully kill yourself. Sometimes the plan is too elaborate, and then there is bound to be a gaffe. When I was a medical student, I had a patient who ate ground glass. He ended up with a lot of severe problems with his stomach and esophagus, but he survived. Then there was the patient who set up an intricate pulley system, hauling a heavy metal engineer's desk up onto the ceiling and sitting underneath it. It didn't kill him, but it did leave him with a lifetime of chronic pain due to the crush injuries. Then there are those brain-injured patients who survive shooting themselves in the head.

It's tougher than you think to end it all, take my word. And after a failed attempt? You thought your life sucked before, just wait.

What is always infinitely hard to predict is the future, when there hasn't yet been an attempt, but there are hints. I can't always tell just how desperate a person is, or how far he'll go to escape his painful life.

Most of us have had friends, family members, or colleagues die at their own hands. How many of us knew it was going to happen? How many of us missed the warning signs, so easy to see in hindsight?

It's easy to blame yourself endlessly when someone you know ends his life. I should've known he was in pain. I should've offered more of my time and my heart. And when it's someone who is assigned to be under your care, it's even easier to beat yourself up.

My first suicide happened when I was a fourth-year resident at the Bronx VA—my last year of training. I was thirty. A thirty-four-year-old guy with a heart of gold—nice guy, but a very sick man with intense mood swings and intermittent psychosis—was assigned to me. This illness is called schizoaffective disorder, and it carries a prognosis more dire than bipolar disorder due to its deteriorating course. When I inherited this patient from the outgoing resident in July, she let me know he was in trouble. I had a talk with him, man to man, my desk in between us. He never took off his dark sunglasses during our discussion. (One of the things I fixated on later, in my own interminable postmortem.)

"You're my most dangerous patient," I began. I assumed he'd like to think of himself in those terms. I could tell by the sunglasses, or so I thought. "You just got out of the hospital after attempting suicide. Statistically, you're at risk to try it again."

He nodded wordlessly. I was hoping he'd start to open up and tell me why, so we could begin to make a connection, but no, just the nodding.

"What can you and I do to keep you alive, I wonder?" I asked. Let him know he's part of the treatment team. We're in this together.

"Search me," he said, shrugging his shoulders.

"Can you please promise me you'll contact me to talk about it if you're feeling suicidal? Can we at least agree on that much?"

"Sure thing, Doc," he promised. He sounded genuine.

Patient contracts for safety, I wrote in his chart.

He seemed to do okay for most of my outpatient year, which goes from July to June, but at some point in the winter, he missed two appointments with me, one for a group session and another for an individual session. After the second missed appointment, I called his wife to see what was up. She told me bluntly that he had checked himself into a hotel, drunk a bottle of vodka, and taken a few months' worth of hoarded prescriptions that I had written for him.

At first I blamed myself, and was nervous that others would blame me as well. If he had hoarded my prescriptions, this meant he was off his meds while I was still seeing him. I was specifically worried about the peer-review process, the morbidity and mortality conference where I would have to present his case to the other doctors and defend my choice of his medications. But then I felt guilty that I was focusing on me, how this reflected badly on my skills as a psychiatrist. I needed to do something to shoulder more of the responsibility, even if the other doctors didn't bear down on me.

I called his widow again, to commiserate. It was a very emotional phone call; I allowed myself to really open up to her loss and grief, and also, most important, to her anger. I needed to feel guilty because I had let both of us down, and she helped me with that, as she had a right to.

She told me how she had known him for eighteen years, and how they'd finally gotten married six months ago. She described how their eight-year-old son kept leaving his seat and going up to the coffin to kiss him good-bye during the open-casket funeral. She shared with me how she felt like his soul had entered her body, and how she spent all day with his ashes, feeling like her heart had been ripped out of her chest and torn apart.

She was full of questions. Why did he leave her so soon after they were finally married? How could he abandon his son? And how could I, his doctor, let this happen?

It was tempting for both of us to blame each other. She asked why I had prescribed certain medications instead of others, and why I couldn't see him more frequently. Wasn't there more I could have done?

I wanted to know why no one thought to call me for help when he stopped talking for a week at home. He began sitting alone in dark rooms, sleeping more and more. Why didn't she let me know what was going on with him? Why didn't he call me?

I didn't realize anything different was happening with him. I fixated on the signs I should've picked up on. He wore his dark sunglasses one day in group therapy. Maybe that meant something. He seemed irritable with the other patients, which was unusual for him. Maybe that should've tipped me off. And why the hell didn't I call him immediately when he missed his first appointment for group therapy?

My patient did not want to be found. He didn't try to hang himself down the hallway while his family ate dinner. He didn't call an ambulance five minutes after he swallowed some pills because he changed his mind. (These are common occurrences in a staged suicidal gesture.) This man checked himself into a hotel room, telling no one where he was going. He left no note, and he took multiple full bottles of multiple medications, chasing the pills down with nearly a quart of vodka. Clearly, he wanted to die and took precautions so that he would not be stopped.

But couldn't I have stopped him anyway?

Mostly, what I heard from other doctors at the VA was how some patients are absolutely intent upon ending their life and we can't always prevent them. That this is a rite of passage. It's a fundamental part of residency training in psychiatry; every doctor loses patients. You learn and grow from it, and you go on to the next patient, trying not to let it happen again.

When I'm at the CPEP deciding whether someone should be kept in the hospital or released, I need to choose the path of least mortality: Will this person go out and kill himself or someone else? Dance in the middle of the FDR and cause an accident? Jump from the Brooklyn Bridge?

My answer, more often than not, is, Who the hell knows? Does anyone see a freakin' crystal ball on my desk? I don't have all the answers. I'm doing the best I can with what I have, which sometimes is not much information at all. I'm always pressured to send the patients out, because we only have so much room at the hospital. The busier we are, the higher my threshold for what gets caught in the safety net, and thus pulled into the safe harbor of the psych ward, such as it is.

There is an element of uncertainty with every T & R. I have to be okay with that ambiguity if I'm going to work weekend after weekend. I trust my gut and try not to gamble too much on any given case, and usually the house wins.

Before I became a psychiatrist, I rationalized that people had a right to commit suicide. If you're at a lousy party, you should be allowed to leave if you're not having a good time. But after talking to that man's widow, I got to experience a fraction of the pain that a suicide causes, and my first time sharing that grief made me see things differently, made me understand more fully my own obligation as a physician.

Suicide is not just about wanting to leave the party. Depression changes the experience, coloring the perception, which makes it impossible to enjoy the party. As a physician, I must combat the illnesses that cause suicidal thoughts and behaviors. I have an obligation to eradicate the depression that poisons the mind, just as surgeons need to defend their patients from the cancers that hijack the body.

Doctors are supposed to alleviate pain. Psychiatrists are meant not only to soothe the despair and hopelessness that a depressed person experiences, but also, I have come to realize, to prevent the pain of the ones who would be left behind. This means I must do all I can to prevent the leaving.

Hole in the River

January 2004. Kathie Russo calls me in the morning on my cell phone, just before I'm leaving the hospital. She should sound frantic, yet her voice is somehow friendly, as always.

"Spalding's missing again."

"Oh, no . . ." I say.

"Can you find out if he's in the ER there, or . . ." she trails off.

The morgue, I think. "Sure. I can ask them if they have any John Does. You want me to call the medical examiner, too?" I ask as casually as I can.

"Yeah. I guess so. I think he's really done it this time. He left on Saturday night, saying he was meeting a friend for dinner, but when he didn't come home I called his friend. He didn't have any plans with him. And Spalding called Theo to say good night around ten o'clock, but he never came back. He left his wallet here."

"Boy, that doesn't sound so good, Kathie, leaving his wallet." I don't say the word: suicide. Spalding has been talking about it for years, and he's made several attempts since I've known him. There was that time on the bridge in Sag Harbor in September of 2002. He didn't jump. That's what EMS calls a "bridge up," as opposed to "bridge down." (There's also a "hang up" and a "cut up," more ways to trivialize the event, surgically removing its gravity.) Then there was another time when he actually did jump off the bridge in October of 2003. And the time he walked into the ocean fully clothed. He's left suicide notes in the past, or a message on the answering machine saying he was going to jump off the Staten Island Ferry. But Kathie says this time there's no note.

"I don't know what to think. All I know is, if he did it, or if he's just pretending he did it . . . I don't think I can do this anymore."

"I know, Kathie. It's horrible, what he's putting you through. And the kids. It's not fair. He's been miserable for such a long time. But I thought he was getting better." Again, I don't say what I'm thinking, which is that it's when depressed people get a little bit better that they finally have the energy and the wherewithal to complete the suicide they've been contemplating. "I'll call the ER and the ME's office and call you back if I find out anything."

I call the AES and ask if they have any unidentified white males in their sixties. They don't, and I dial the city morgue next. They're on the next block, just north of Bellevue, and I'm tempted to walk over there. It's probably easier than getting someone to pick up the phone, if it's anything like Bellevue. I'm placed on hold, and I really have to pee. I dance around my office with the phone cradled in my neck. I'm six months pregnant now, so I have to use the bathroom every few hours at least. It's hard not to think about Spalding's kids while I'm waiting. I imagine they're all sitting around, watching the door, hoping he's going to walk in so everything can go back to the way it was before.

Only it hasn't been the way it was for years. Kathie has been through hell dealing with Spalding's depressions, and there have been a handful of phone calls to me along the way, especially since his car accident in Ireland the summer before 9/11. He had two psychiatric hospitalizations in 2002, the first at Silver Hill in June and then at Cornell in September. The Cornell admission lasted for months and months. I remember Kathie calling me to complain how she couldn't get them to release him, because Spalding wouldn't tell them he wasn't suicidal anymore. Basically, he was, and he didn't know enough to lie. I bet his Cornell psychiatrist knew what a lot of us pushed to the back of our minds: He was absolutely going to kill himself eventually.

For the next few weeks, I drive home on Sunday and Monday mornings, my car covered with snow, heading north on the FDR, the East River on my right. Spalding's out there somewhere, I think as I glance at the ice. If he did jump off the Staten Island Ferry, then his body is most likely in the East River because of the currents. And all the evidence is pointing to the Staten Island Ferry. The call to Theo came from the ter-

minal there. Someone who works on the ferry reported that they saw
him the night before, on Friday night, when he placed his wallet on the
bench and walked over to the boat's railing. Maybe it was a dry run, or
maybe he just wasn't quite ready, but I'm afraid he did jump into the
river the next night. The police tell Kathie that his body will probably
turn up in the spring, when the ice thaws. I think about that every time
I drive home.

It's odd to think of him drowning. He'd have to purposely try not to
swim. All of his suicide attempts involved water, jumping off of bridges,
walking into the ocean, letting his sailboat drag him while he hung onto
the rudder. I don't know why it had to be in the water, but it seemed
like it was crucial to him. I know he can swim; I've gone swimming
with him up at our lake house. Right after I got married in the summer
of 1999, Spalding and his two sons came by for the afternoon. Theo,
who was probably four back then, jumped off the dock over and over
again, wearing a swimsuit with built-in Styrofoam floaters. I picked up
Kathie at the train and we all had dinner. I remember that we talked
about JFK Jr. That was the day they found his body.

A few summers later, we went to visit them at their lake house. Molly
was three. I had taken her to three lakes in three days, but Spalding's
lake was by far the best. I remember how crystal clear the water was,
and how the fish swam right up to us, unafraid. We sat with Spalding
on the shore, but it didn't seem like him anymore. He had changed so
much since the car accident. He was silent, morose, horribly depressed.
The neighbors came by to say hello and Kathie did most of the talking.
I remember wondering if he was aware of how elderly and frail he appeared. When he went out on the deck to start the fire for dinner, he
tripped on the bag of charcoal. He was having a harder time walking
because of his foot drop, a result of the accident. None of us said anything, but my heart lurched as his body did. He had aged so much in
two years.

I should've thought that there was a connection between the car accident and his depression, but it never occurred to me. Spalding had
such a complicated picture: a lifetime of obsessive neurosis and exis-
tential angst, which blossomed over time into something that looked
more like bipolar disorder. After the car accident, his symptoms became much more intense, and I should have realized that he had a head
injury in his frontal lobe, and that this was the likely culprit causing

his psychiatric symptoms. Maybe if he had come to me as a patient in my office instead of talking to me as a friend, I would've been able to pull back and see the big picture. But I had been reluctant to treat him, referring him to a colleague instead. It was only when Spalding saw Oliver Sacks later in the fall and gave him his whole history that the decision was made to put him on Lamictal, a mood stabilizer that is more appropriate for head injuries than many of the other medications that had failed to bring him back around.

And then for a while it seemed that he was doing much better. He was working on a new monologue about the accident and its resultant depression. But somehow it just wasn't enough. He was still hell-bent on drowning. That Saturday, before he jumped off the ferry, he saw the movie *Big Fish* with his sons at the theater right around the corner from my office. At the end of the movie, the father goes into the ocean, turns into a fish, and swims away. Maybe Spalding decided that film had finally given him permission, or he wanted the boys to see it to understand what he was planning.

In early March, when the ice thaws, Spalding's body turns up on the shoreline in Brooklyn, and it is as if he has died a fourth time, after the car accident, the debilitating depression, and the presumed suicide.

Jeremy and I go to the memorial at Lincoln Center; it is standing room only. Kathie has done a great job organizing a dazzling turnout of eulogizers. Spalding was, above all else, an amazing storyteller, and it is a fitting tribute to him that the evening is full of entertaining tales of his talent as well as his titanic struggle with depression. There is just the right balance of laughter and tears.

It is nine days before Jojo is born, April 13, 2004. I am ungainly, as I was when I danced with Spalding at the *Harper's* party the night before I gave birth to Molly. I am glad I get to see Kathie again, before the delivery, and to feel Spalding's presence again for a moment before my second child is born. It feels like a blessing, somehow.

God Put a Smile Upon Your Face

Monday morning and I have twenty minutes until sign-out. I waddle to the coffee shop to pick up my breakfast, walking through the ambulance bay. It's a busy morning in the AES and there are three stretchers waiting to be triaged, each with two EMS workers in attendance. A drunken, gray-haired man with a bloody nose, his face red and raw from the sun, is telling his female ambulance driver, "I don't usually look this bad, you know," as if he's hoping there's a chance he can ask her out.

"I know you don't, sweetie," she soothes.

There is a large woman on a stretcher, her shirt open, the dark hairs leading to her pelvis exposed. She is talking loudly, rapidly into her cell phone, "I was up all night working on my screenplay. You know the one Spielberg's directing?" With a short wave, I get the triage nurse's attention as I am walking by. "This one's ours," I mouth, and smile. She smiles back and nods vigorously. Evidently, she's figured that out too.

As I return to the CPEP with my brown paper bags full of breakfast, the screenwriter has already made her way to our area. She is sitting on one of the green interconnected bucket seats, still talking on her phone, which she won't hand over to the hospital police officer. He asks her again, and she states imperiously, "Do you mind? I'm talking to my agent!" and then hisses into the phone, "I said, I'm at Bellevue. Come down and get me out of here, now!"

The HP tries to explain the no cell phone policy, and so she turns to leave, saying, "Okay, then. I'll use my phone outside."

I interrupt, and explain to her that she needs to stay to be evaluated. "Since you were brought here by ambulance, you can't leave this area until you're seen by a psychiatrist." I have lain down the gauntlet.

"Are you from West Virginia?" she asks me, out of nowhere.

"No," I reply. "Why?"

"They do a lot of inbreeding down there."

I stare at her dumbly.

Zing.

I break into a wide grin, score one for her in the air with my finger, and spin around on my clogs. She's not going to be my problem today. I'm getting ready to sign out, saving her for the day staff. Ahhh, shift work.

I take my breakfast into the nurses' station, and set up my food before we do sign-out rounds. The phone rings. It is my pal Dr. Robert, an attending from the inpatient wards who occasionally moonlights in the CPEP. He calls everyone "baby." (I have another Bellevue friend who calls everyone "lovey.") I think it's cute. Moreover, I think he's cute. Before I met Jeremy, he was my number-one Bellevue crush. Especially when he would come into work on his Rollerblades. He actually skated through the hospital to get to the CPEP. I loved that.

"Julie, baby, how are you?" he says, sounding like a Hollywood agent.

"Great, I'm as big as a house and I pee every two seconds. I'm going out on maternity leave any day now, taking four months off, not that it pays. You'll think of me while you're working, I hope? All summer, I mean?"

He takes it in stride, barely skipping a beat. "Oh, you . . . Of course, of course. Listen, can you sign out something for me this morning? Make sure Maxwell hears it, okay? We've been having a lot of problems up here the past few weeks, and I keep forgetting to tell you guys."

"What is it?" I ask.

"You gotta only send us 'bloods,' or 'crips,' not both."

"Come on, really?"

"No, I'm totally serious! We're having like mini gang-wars up here."

"You think we should designate your ward as a 'crip' ward and we can do 18 North as a 'blood' ward?"

"Whatever it takes, but I'm telling you, it's for real. Only bloods or crips. Not both. Sign it out."

"Okay, boss," I say, getting ready to hang up. I have no idea how true those words will become. After I leave Bellevue, he'll become the next director of CPEP, the third replacement since Lucy died.

When I Get Home

I deliver Jojo even more rapidly than Molly. He is pushed out just twenty minutes after arriving at Mount Sinai. He has an old-soul look in his eyes, and his face resembles nothing as much as a squished-up elderly man, more from Jeremy's side of the family than mine. I spend the first few days feeling like I'm nursing my father-in-law.

I take the summer off from work, and the four of us spend most of it on Cape Cod. By the end of August, I am dying to return to the hospital.

"I can't wait 'til I can get back to Bellevue and have a little peace and quiet," I say to my friends. The irony of deeming CPEP a calm oasis is not lost on me or anyone else. "At least there, I'm the boss," I explain. "When I ask someone to do something, it gets done. They don't whine or throw a tantrum. Or, if they do, at least I can medicate and restrain them," I joke.

I find I'm losing my patience easily with Molly these days. She is reacting to a new baby in the house by testing limits, defying my authority (such as it is), and being oppositional on a daily basis. I remember one of my patients in my private practice warning me when I mentioned her age, "You know, everyone talks about the terrible twos, but no one warns you about the fucking fours!" I take solace as I hear from mother after mother that four is a particularly difficult age, a miniature adolescence full of rebellion and drama. At one point, we are wrestling on the sand in front of the beach house as I whisper harshly into her ear, "I am in charge. You are not in charge." I am eager to go somewhere where I can have more control over my environment.

It is September of 2004 when I return to CPEP. As I walk through the ambulance bay doors, I'm so overwhelmed by a sense of homecoming that I can practically smell the turkey. I bring pictures of the kids, and the nurses are appropriately appreciative of their good looks, and they make sure to tell me how thin I look, God bless them.

And then there's Chuck, who has always made fun of how big my butt is, whether I was eating for two or not. When I was pregnant the first time around, he would measure the width of it and then record it on the wall under the clock. Using a long envelope typically used to store chest X-rays, he would hold it up behind me when I wasn't looking and then mark off my dimensions, making two little blue pen marks on the glossy beige surface of the wall. When I get back from maternity leave, despite the nurses' compliments, he remeasures and compares the width to show me it actually isn't any smaller. *Thanks, pal. Maybe we can paint these walls sometime soon?*

"Julie, we are so glad you are back here with us." Nancy's beefy arms open warmly to greet me.

"I don't know, Nance. It's been a while. It may take me a bit to get back up to speed." I am particularly worried about the computer, entering orders and retrieving data. Do I remember my password, or the cumbersome twenty steps necessary to enter an order for a chest X-ray?

"Oh, it's just like riding a bicycle. You never forget. You'll be T-and-R-ing like the best of 'em in no time," she assures me.

I look out the triage window and see some neatly groomed men, all dressed alike.

"Looks like an FBI case is coming in. See those blue jackets? And those haircuts! These guys are like clones!" I walk out to investigate.

"Good evening," I say, welcoming the men to my home away from home. "I'm Doctor Holland. What'd you bring me?"

"Mr. Rocket Scientist here thought he'd build himself a pipe bomb. He was barricaded up inside a makeshift structure with the bomb. We're not sure if he was trying to kill himself or take a lot of people out with him."

"Oh, and I didn't get you anything!" I joke with the G-man. It's my oldest bit, well-worn from years of triage banter, and it feels good to slip back into it like a favorite sweatshirt. The federal agent, against his better judgment, cracks a smile.

Rita registers the patient and asks for the old chart. When it arrives, I see he's got a history of a few prior suicide attempts. Once, he overdosed on drugs and was in a coma for several weeks. Another time he shot himself in the chest with a nail gun, requiring surgery. The second one is the red flag. I spend the next ten minutes lecturing the medical student on what sorts of things should make you think of psychosis instead of garden-variety depression when you evaluate suicide attempts.

"People who stab themselves or create elaborate devices to kill themselves are more likely to be psychotic than those who overdose on pills, slit their wrists, or hang themselves," I explain. "In general, the crazier they are, the more bizarre and unreliable their suicide plans."

Our suicidal bomber needs to be evaluated, per the FBI, to make sure he isn't homicidal. I spend some time with him, allowing the medical student to ask most of the questions. After he details how he spent three months constructing the barricade to assure that no one else would be hurt in the explosion, I know the FBI can go.

Once I've tucked away the bomber, I meet my next patient, a Trump Tower trust-fund guy who's staying at the Plaza while they work on some water damage in his apartment. I don't know what it is about the Plaza Hotel, but they sure end up sending us a lot of business. They might as well have a CPEP shuttle for their guests. People in a manic phase of bipolar illness will go there and hole up for weeks on end, burning through tens of thousands of dollars as they get more out of control. Other folks will check in there prior to suicide attempts. The Plaza is a classy joint, and I guess some people prefer opulent surroundings just before they end up at Bellevue. Most important, it turns out rich people can go crazy too. Being loaded doesn't insulate you from mental illness. You can come from the Port Authority bus terminal, or you can come from Trump Tower. Bellevue, like insanity itself, is the great equalizer.

This particular patient has a wealthy family in the art world, and when he's psychiatrically stable, he is the manager of an art gallery. Because of his long history with psychotic illness, he often can't work. Once I get on the phone with the family, I get a better understanding of what "water damage" really means: He's been hoarding his urine and feces in plastic garbage bags throughout his condominium, and it has started to damage some of the fine art he is collecting and storing there. I don't know why people collect and catalogue their excretions, but it happens. A lot. Maybe the toilet becomes terrifying when you're psychotic, or maybe the collection business is an indicator of extreme obsessiveness, an irrational unwillingness to let go of anything.

Luckily, the family has intervened in time, and while the "water" did damage some costly pieces, many other works have been salvaged. He is admitted voluntarily so that we can get him back on his medications. My assumption is that he will be transferred to a different, cushier hospital once he calms down a bit.

The other interesting patient of the night, in keeping with the "money can't buy happiness" theme, is a young woman with what looks to be a $30,000 ring on her hand. The dark mother-of-pearl stone, nearly an inch in diameter, is surrounded by diamonds. She has been heartbroken, she tells the triage nurse, since her mother died aboard one of the planes on 9/11. We are still seeing fallout from the attack, although the three-year mark is next week. Anniversary reactions are very common in trauma. I have been encouraging my patients to try to leave the television off as 9/11 approaches. The people who have been doing better will often have a resurgence of mourning and its attendant melancholia as the media reminds us all of what happened.

Some of the people who took 9/11 the hardest have only gotten worse over time. The reminders of that day are still too prevalent, and terrorism is a potent weapon against mental health. There has been a constant hum of anxiety in the city since the collapse of the twin towers. Our government won't let us forget we're in danger; New Yorkers are still on guard against the fear of loss which never fully abated after the attacks. Everyone has been taking psych meds or martinis to cope.

Many people fell off the wagon after 9/11, especially the cops and the firefighters. EMS was not bringing survivors from the towers, they were bringing us drunks. I remember Daniel complaining about it in rounds one morning that September, but I spoke up, since I'm supposed to be the substance abuse expert at CPEP. "These people need our assistance just like any other victims of the attack."

The gal with the ring has been admitted to our EOU. She's been depressed and drinking for years since her mom died, and now she's talking about suicide. She was on the phone with her friend in Florida when she let on that she had cut her wrist. The friend called 911 in New York City and now my new patient—perfectly coiffed, nicely dressed, with an air of supreme entitlement, yet carrying a teddy bear—has every family member and friend calling us on her behalf to get her out of Bellevue. The family arranges for her to go to a private uptown hospital, but her insurance office is closed over the weekend. I call Columbia psych ER, and they are willing to accept the transfer, unbelievably, without insurance verification because of some guarantee made by the family.

Now all I have to do is secure the ambulance transfer from Bellevue to Columbia without an insurance authorization, which means a family member has to give a credit card number. I am on the phone with a friend of hers in New York City, who refers to Bellevue as a "snake pit," then says, "Nothing personal, I mean you working there and all, but we gotta get her outta there." The brother in California is on the phone bitching about paying for the ambulance, feeling it's the hospital's responsibility, but Bellevue doesn't typically pay for transfers, unless it's to another city hospital because we're full. Usually the patient's insurance company pays for a transfer. The only other option is that she spend the weekend in CPEP, which nobody wants, except maybe the cheap brother.

The staff wants this gal to go—she is issuing one demand after another—and I want one less patient in the area if Columbia is willing to accept the transfer. Finally, the brother and the ambulance company are connected so he can give them his credit card information, but all he has is American Express, which this ambulance company doesn't take. I have to call around to find an ambulance company that does, and the staff are cracking jokes left and right.

Rita says, giggling, "When your suicidal sister is stuck at Bellevue, don't forget your VISA card, 'cause the transfer won't go through with American Express."

I reply, "Having a MasterCard to get your girl outa that snake pit . . . priceless."

It feels so good to be back, I can hardly stand it. I love Chuck and Nancy, and Rita and Vera, and all the other staff at CPEP, and I am home again.

But for how long? And how soon until the burnout creeps back in?

Beautiful Boy

I'm wiped out from the kids at home and was hoping to turn in early tonight, but it is not to be. I'm staying up to wait for a pre-arraignment evaluation that's being transferred to us. A Bronx hospital called earlier about a psychotic prisoner they thought we should admit to our forensic unit. He's hearing the voice of a man who he says protects him, a man he calls "Chance."

I start with my usual—ignore the perp and ask the cop, "What's the charge?"

"Endangering the welfare of a child," he answers. "It'll be Murder One as soon as they take the kid off life support. He beat up his baby. Pretty bad. I doubt the kid's gonna make it."

"How old's the kid?" I ask.

"Ten months," the cop says.

I try to play it cool, like it doesn't faze me.

"I don't know which are worse, the baby-killers or the mother-rapers." I want him to think I've seen it all. And maybe by now I have? When I was a medical student I did see one patient who had raped his mother— totally psychotic, of course—the only thing I can think of as horrific as killing a baby. I have now seen two of each in the seventeen years since I entered medical school, but I toss it off to the cop like this is standard stuff, no big deal.

And then I stop to think: He probably doesn't see this all the time either. We're both acting nonchalant, business as usual, and we should know better; it's a very big deal.

Nancy and I decide to see the patient together. Usually the nurse triages the patient first, and then the doctor does the second evaluation, but it's a very busy night and we're both wiped out; we streamline the process to keep things moving.

We sit side by side in the triage room to do the interview, our paperwork in front of us. The patient/prisoner is a surprisingly good-looking guy, with medium-length dreadlocks and light brown skin. He sustains good eye contact and his voice is soft. Nancy asks him why he's been arrested, and he starts off telling us some obscure detail about his son's current medical status.

"My boy's intestines are perforated, or something like that."

"Well . . . how'd that happen?" I ask.

"I beat my baby up," he says, looking stunned. "He wouldn't stop crying and so I punched him over and over." His eyes plead with me, and I can see that he is completely unhinged, but he's working to bury it. Nancy wants to know where the mother was during this time, and he tells her she was in the next room watching TV. "She never helps with the baby. I have to do everything: the Pampers, the bottles. And she won't tell me how to calm him down. She knows the secret way and she won't tell me."

All of this is hitting way too close to home for me, and Nancy knows it. She looks over at me, gauging my response, and I cock my head, shrug my shoulders. I don't know what I'm trying to communicate to her. I'm okay with proceeding, I guess. I have a nine-and-a-half-month-old baby boy at home and this guy's son is ten months old. Diapers, bottles, crying, calming . . . we have everything in common, and I can feel myself getting sucked in. And the mom having a secret magic trick to calm the baby holds true in our household because I am nursing.

"Is she nursing? The baby's mother?" I ask.

"No," he answers simply, then adds, "She's my wife. I only married her because she was pregnant."

He is answering questions clearly, succinctly, but later in the interview, he explains that he's been hearing voices most of his life. "The cocaine sometimes calms them down," he tells us. He is smoking a lot of crack, and blunts with pot and crack in them. So is his wife. The prisoner tells me how his own mother used to punish him by locking him in a closet when he was a kid, and how this imaginary friend, "Chance," used to appear and take care of him, talk to him. Chance has been talking to him ever since.

I can't figure out if he's a schizophrenic or not. Maybe his mother's sadism caused him to fall apart. A severely stressful childhood can put anyone over the edge; their personality structure shatters, and they may develop alternate personalities. Not everyone who hears voices has the full-blown syndrome of schizophrenia. The chronic cocaine use could bring on hallucinations as well, especially in someone with psychotic tendencies.

He tells me he's been diagnosed as schizophrenic in the past. My gut tells me he's too well-related (he connects easily on an emotional level) and organized, but other psychiatrists have disagreed. He's been tried on several different antipsychotics, but he never makes it to his follow-up appointments and eventually stops taking his meds.

He says he's hallucinating now, and the transfer paperwork from the other hospital is making a good case for that as well, though he doesn't appear to be responding to internal stimuli. Psychosis aside, I need to determine if he'll be safe when he's alone in a cell. He doesn't volunteer anything suicidal-sounding until the last second, when we are done talking, as the cop pulls his wheelchair out of the interview room.

"It shoulda been me," he says softly.

I know what he's getting at.

I also know that Nancy wants him out. We're full to the brim with patients and prisoners, and she doesn't think he's going to do it. I usually try to appease Nancy in these situations. She's the nurse in charge and we usually happily agree on what to do with all the patients. I bite my tongue and start the paperwork to release him back to the police, dancing around any words that might allude to dangerousness necessitating a psychiatric admission.

I try to talk the cop into taking him back to be arraigned. It's a hard sell, maybe the hardest one I've ever had to make for a prisoner T & R. I'm doing my best, but the cop is nervous. I am having very real fantasies of this guy hanging himself with his shirt in a holding cell somewhere, left alone for five minutes too long. I think this officer is having the same fears. The cop sees what I see: Some part of this guy knows how massively he just screwed up. "It shoulda been me." If he really believes it, I know he'll have the desire, and quite possibly the means, to carry it out while waiting in a cell.

Obviously the patient has poor impulse control. He beat up his baby. What makes me think he's not going to turn his rage on himself next? I don't tell Nancy I'm having second thoughts. I want the night to go smoothly, and it always goes better if I don't go up against her. The problem is, now I'm going up against my intuition, and I know I shouldn't do that, either.

Luckily, the cop gives me an out. I can blame it on him. "I really don't feel comfortable taking this guy back to booking, Doc. I got a funny feeling about this one."

I walk into the nurses' station looking defeated. "NYPD won't take this guy, Nancy. We gotta eat it."

A few minutes later, the cop asks me to interview him again. "Uh, listen, Doc. I think you better talk with this guy some more. He just told me he's planning on hanging himself in the cell."

Just what we were afraid of.

I wheel the prisoner back into the triage room. I was hoping that since he didn't volunteer any suicidal thoughts during our first superficial, controlled interview, I could document it as such and get on with my night. But now we're going to get into it. And of course, like rubbing my tongue against a canker sore to see if it still hurts, I can't stop myself. I decide to go for it whole hog, diving in. I might as well learn as much as I can about what makes a man beat his own son to death. One of the perks of the job, I'll confess to my friends later. "You read the cover of the *Post,* about these crazy people committing heinous crimes, and you think, *What kind of man could possibly do that?* I have the pleasure of meeting these men and trying to answer that question."

But I am growing weary, as time goes by, of these golden opportunities. It doesn't feel like such a gift anymore, getting to see the underbelly of humanity. I'm starting to think that maybe I want to live in the sanitized, Upper-East-Side version of New York City, knee-deep in denial, seeing the good in people all around me. I'm afraid that the longer I work at Bellevue, the harder it will be to revert to being oblivious. It's like cooking an egg: it can never go back to soft-boiled once it's hard-boiled.

All this exposure to the depravity, to man's inhumanity to man, I'm frightened that I won't be able to walk away from it, forget it, and get on with my life. I'll never again be the person standing at the edge of the subway platform waiting for a train, instead of leaning up against the wall so no one can push me onto the rails just as the train pulls into the station. I'll never walk by the Empire State Building without thinking about the shooter who took out so many people. I'll never run around the lake in Central Park without thinking of the "Baby-Faced Butcher," the young altar boy so incapacitated by the combination of his psych meds and malt liquor that he gutted a man and dumped him in the pond.

I'm also never going to be able to stop worrying that one of my children will end up with a debilitating psychiatric disorder. I've shared that pain with too many parents, and I am now terrified that this will eventually become my pain as well.

I have a growing sense that I need to do something before I become irreversibly hard-boiled, in a last-ditch effort to protect my newly expanding rich, warm, liquid center. Like the body walling off an abscess with layers of scar tissue, my callous demeanor protects and defends my tender interior. But I don't want to lose touch completely with my softer parts, which help to make me a better doctor and an emotionally attuned mother.

I think I'm going to have to get out of Bellevue. Soon.

It should've been me." This is known in psychiatry as the doorknob statement. Named for the timing of its delivery, it is the baited hook dangled at the end of the therapeutic hour, just as the patient is leaving the office with his hand on the door. Seasoned shrinks know that those things mentioned as the patient is leaving the room are often the most important things they will ever say, the things they don't really want to give up. On the other hand, doorknob statements can be a well-timed manipulative ploy. The patient knows his time is up but wants more, wants to create drama, to test you to see if you'll continue to be his audience or shoo him out the door for the next patient. But somehow,

this isn't one of those times. He isn't one of those people.

g down and needs somewhere to land.

, this baby-killer, is still somehow a sympathetic character to me. On some level, I am drawn to him. Perhaps it is as simple as a physical attraction—his charisma, his pheromones—but mostly I think what's going on is he's playing into my rescue fantasies. I want to help him, to catch him as he's falling. If nothing else, we are both parents; at least I can connect with him on that level. From his perspective, he has no reason to align with me, a psychiatrist. He's been psychotic since childhood with inadequate psychiatric care. No one's rescued him yet, why trust me now?

Maybe he knows that I decide whether he goes to prison or upstairs. Maybe he knows that it's cushier in the forensic unit, and if he can convince the doctor he's in danger, he'll be admitted instead of sent to arraignment. Maybe, but I doubt it. Not this time. This guy's for real.

He tells me his wife is using just as much cocaine as he is, and he complains, the way my girlfriends complain about their husbands, that she is not pulling her weight in the child-care department. He has to do everything when he gets home—change the baby, wash the bottles. He keeps mentioning how he had just gotten home from doing his taxes. I wish he would stop saying that. Normal people have meetings with accountants and figure out how much they owe the government. Why is this baby-killer saying that? And why is he speaking my language of housewifery, child care, and martyrdom? When he again mentions the secret mommy way of calming the baby, he makes me feel guilty, like I am his wife, and I should've shown him how to calm down our son. It's my fault for pulling that power play.

"I'm the one who has to get up in the morning with him and give him a bottle and put him down in front of the TV." Great. Now I've got a visual. Why does he have to give me an image of a little boy in a diaper plopped in front of *Barney* or *Teletubbies*? An innocent little boy who is as good as dead, beaten to death by his father, who was once an innocent little boy abused by his mother, who was once . . .

"He just wouldn't stop whining. I hit him and yelled at him to stop crying, and he still wouldn't stop crying."

I know about the exquisite frustration at the whining, or when you can't make the crying stop. When Jojo had colic, and the crying was ceaseless, I marveled at how any parent could cope with it, why more children weren't hurt by their caretakers. Sometimes parenting seems like the most difficult job there is. Because I've come to see firsthand how abusing a child causes a lifetime of psychic pain and psychiatric illness, I'm able to sympathize with this patient. He has failed his obligations as a parent, obviously, in the most extreme way imaginable, but what he has done is not beyond my imagining.

"It'd make sense if I die after what I did to him," he cries. "It'd balance things. So then I can die and he can live."

Bingo.

There's the psychosis—he thinks he can bring his son back to life by killing himself. He's tipping some delusional scale of justice. And even if he's not crazy, he still knows he should die for what he's done, and he's prepared to make that happen.

Either way, he's not safe to be alone in a cell.

I let him know we're going to keep him here in the hospital. "We're going to try to help you. I'm going to start some medicine so Chance's voice will get a little softer at least. Maybe it'll go away entirely. And we'll keep you on a watch so you can't hurt yourself. Okay?"

"Okay," he says simply, relieved. He sobs quietly in his high-backed wheelchair, his wrist cuffed to its wooden arm.

He eventually goes up to the forensic psychiatry unit, admitted as an involuntary patient as are all forensic cases, but I can't get him out of my head for days and days. I finally call up to the prison ward a few days later to find out which doctor got assigned to him. It's my friend Rose, and I'm glad that she's open to my need to debrief.

"I know! That guy totally got to me, too!" she confides. She's not sure what to make of him either. "I opted to take him at face value, so I continued the Risperdal you started."

"Oh, that's good. That makes me feel better, actually," I admit.

"They're both pretty heavy-duty cocaine addicts, he and his wife. They spend most of their checks early in the month on drugs, and then they don't have enough left over for diapers and formula."

"Lovely."

"And here's the best part, are you ready?" she asks. "The wife is pregnant again. Three months. She wants to keep it."

"Oh man, Rose . . . I honestly don't know how much more of this I can take."

A Hard Day's Night

One Sunday night I go to a cocktail party before work. I have a glass of wine, and half of another. By the time I get to the hospital, my cheeks are a bit pink, and I'm all smiley, glassy-eyed.

When I roll into the triage area, Rita smiles right back at me.

"Don't you look happy? Sorry to tell you, but it's a disaster in here. If you're smart, you'll back away quietly . . . go home. We never saw you."

"You so funny!" I say, laughing as I go in.

Big mistake. Shoulda backed away. Worst Night Ever.

EMS just keeps bringing 'em in and bringing 'em in and each one is crazier than the last. Even the walk-ins have incredibly heartbreaking tales. I can't discharge anyone, and the bodies keep piling up.

Doctors talk about the patients on their service in terms of how many they are "carrying," and what their "patient load" is. This is no misnomer. The more patients you are responsible for, the heavier your burden.

I thought that I would be able to order in a nice meal and sit down to something tasty around eight or nine p.m. No matter how busy it is, I usually find time to eat some sushi, or Thai food, or at least a coffee shop salad. Tonight, I don't stop to take a breath, and it's past one in the morning before I'm finally eating a Bellevue baloney sandwich that I fished out of the fridge.

The resident is doing the best she can to stay above water, but she doesn't have as many helpers as usual. There is only one medical student to assist instead of the usual three or four. Also, it's the medical student's first time down here and she's nervous. Normally during their first time in the ER, the medical students just shadow a resident, sitting in on interviews but not asking many questions, and not writing up any charts. Tonight, this cannot be. It's baptism by fire and I send the medical student on her own to see cases. "I need all hands on deck," I apologize. "I'm going to have you see a case or two on your own. No one too psychotic or dangerous, though, don't worry. I'll try to pick someone with a story to tell."

Luckily, there are plenty of patients in need of a shoulder to cry on. They'll keep her busy and I know she'll be safe. It's important to match the medical students up with a patient who will be educational but nonviolent. That way, when they're done talking, I can do a little teaching. I can explain why someone is acting a certain way, or how their medicines aren't working, or how their street drugs of choice *are* working. There won't be much time for teaching tonight, but I can at least make sure the student gets interesting, talkative patients who won't try to strangle her.

The detainable area is packed with patients who are done being processed, but we have nowhere to send any of them. The up-wards are completely full. The forensic ward, which is hardly ever full, has been backed up all weekend. We have multiple prisoners who need to be admitted, each of them trailing two cops, and the CPEP looks like a precinct. Again.

Not only are we chock-full of prisoners and their police escorts, but tonight, these particular patients are more medically complicated than usual. Typically, the police cases are healthy at the physical level. They are young sociopaths on minimal medications with few medical problems. But not on the Worst Night Ever.

The prisoner who just stabbed his wife has a broken leg, which was casted in the medical ER. To further complicate his medical picture, he has a number of fresh cuts on his head, which is shaved because he recently had a brain tumor removed. Oh yeah, and he also has leukemia. Plus, he is totally out of his mind, yelling about the apocalypse, and it's difficult to sedate him due to the head injury/brain tumor situation. People with neurological disorders tend to get disinhibited when they're sedated, sort of like a loud drunk. He's doing his part to add to the noise level in the area, making it feel even more chaotic.

Another prisoner is a very thin, sick-looking gentleman with long-standing AIDS and hepatitis C. On top of that, he has recently been diagnosed with lung cancer. He told his stepson he was going to kill him and his mother with a revolver, but then he decided to turn the gun on himself instead. No one was shot, thanks to the kid tackling his stepfather, but the patient ended up running into the street as soon as he freed himself. He was eventually caught, subdued, and brought in by EMS, the stepson riding along in the rig to help calm him.

But he's far from calm. In the nondetainable area, when our hospital police remove his shoelaces and belt, the patient tries to stab himself in the neck with his belt buckle. This gentleman "isn't going anywhere but up," as we say. Because he's arrested, he must be accepted onto the forensics unit. And the divas running 19 West tell us when they can and cannot accept admissions. This whole weekend, it's been more on the cannot side of things. So we wait.

I've also got a female prisoner doing anything she can think of to get herself admitted and therefore transferred to Elmhurst. First she threatens, in a general way, that she is going to hurt herself. Then she tells us she's pregnant. Finally, she goes into the bathroom (her police escort stands outside the door instead of going in with her) and tries to stab herself in the genitals with a pen, saying she's giving herself an abortion. She comes out of the bathroom to show us her bloody panties. We can't tell if she is bleeding because she has her period and therefore isn't pregnant, or if it's because she has just pierced her own flesh, or if she has actually aborted her fetus. But we're just too busy tonight. The bar has been set incredibly high for admissions, and she isn't quite making it over. If she goes to Elmhurst, we still have to keep her for hours to medically clear her. We decide to discharge her via the medical ER so they can have a look and see if she has done any permanent damage to herself or her unborn baby—if there even *is* a baby.

We are sending out everybody that we possibly can, but it is busier, crazier, and more jam-packed with patients than I've ever seen. I am starting to turn people away at the door.

"Sorry, but we're not seeing any walk-ins tonight," I tell them as they try to come in. I've never done that before. It goes against everything Bellevue stands for, and everything I believe in, but tonight my beliefs are changing. Usually, it's "Give us your sick, your tired, your poor," but tonight it's "Go tell it to Beth Israel. We're full."

After a quick evaluation, we even send out a woman brought in by EMS from an apartment building where, according to her boyfriend, she was "swinging out the window like she was on a jungle gym." She had walked into his apartment and seen him in the shower having sex with another woman. She tried to jump out the window (dramatically, making a scene in front of the naked couple) but the boyfriend pulled her back in. It sounds like total theatrics to me, though, and he agrees that she probably wasn't really going to hurt herself. The patient is pre-occupied with an exam she has to get home and study for, which makes me think she probably isn't planning on doing herself in anytime soon. Normally, with a story that sounds this dangerous, we'd hold her over-night for observation, but not tonight. Too many people, nowhere to put any of them, and I'm feeling braver about discharging patients than I've ever felt, because now I'm counting down the days until I leave this nuthouse.

"What are they gonna do, fire me?" is a well-worn refrain by now. It is late winter, and I've made my decision. I aim to be out of here by July first. The medical new year can be rung in without me; I am mov-ing on, saving what's left of myself. Head for the lifeboats! Women and children first!

The night is crammed full of dismal stories and dejected people. One twentysomething gal called 911 saying she was afraid she was hav-ing a nervous breakdown. Her boyfriend of eighteen months had taken her to some man's apartment in Queens to have sex with the guy for money. They all hung out and smoked crack and then the trick paid her boyfriend $150, so he split with the money. Later, when she finally tracked the boyfriend down, he broke up with her because she was a whore. She didn't know whether she wanted to kill him or herself. Then she tells us the only thing that's keeping her from ending her life is that she's pregnant . . . again. Okay, so she couldn't stop smoking crack dur-ing her last pregnancy and she lost the twins at five months, but this time she is planning on stopping before her second trimester. Only she's already sixteen weeks.

The medical student is recounting her past history. "She was gang-raped at twelve and has been prostituting herself ever since. She over-dosed on pills after the trauma at age twelve and again at age seventeen."

Her life story sounds horrendous. She has two children from two different fathers. One is staying with the baby's father and the other is with the baby's paternal grandmother. She has become addicted to crack somewhere along the way, and at this point she mostly prostitutes herself to support her habit, which means she isn't really saving up any of her earnings. She is a "crack whore," for lack of better words, though this is a pejorative term that doesn't begin to convey the misery it should, and she's had a miserable existence since puberty. The weird thing is, she looks pretty well put together and is actually sort of charming. She is very, very smiley—telling us her horrible life story and smiling, smiling, smiling.

"Maybe I can just stay for a few days to get my shit together?" she asks sweetly. We decide she is in complete denial, in total disconnect with how intensely miserable her life is, and it's probably healthier that way. We let her stay.

I've just finished hearing about another case and I tell the resident he needs to discharge the patient. He looks at me as if I am a monster.

"I don't know if you've ever heard me say this before," I tell him, "but all of it is sad, so none of it is sad." This is a line I often use with the medical students and residents when they try to convince me how pitiable a patient's situation is. "What I mean is, I have to set the bar high—my threshold for what will get to me, what reaches me—because all I hear is horribly sad stories every shift I work."

I've been working at Bellevue for nearly nine years now. Because it takes more to break through and touch me, I will discharge patients that other doctors would surely keep. This frequently offends the medical students I am working with, and the residents as well. I know they think I am too harsh, unfeeling. I have a reputation for being callous and uncaring. It's all a front, of course, and one that I'm having a harder and harder time maintaining, but they don't seem to get that. Lousy shrinks, I guess.

"The first casualty of life at CPEP is a sympathetic ear," I continue. "You stay down here long enough and you'll learn that you need to look beyond the story to the question of danger." I try to soften my tone. I am here to teach, not to be defensive about my hardened demeanor. "The bottom line is, is it safe to release the patient? Will they kill themselves, or take out someone else? I factor their miserable childhood into the equation, yes, but usually that's extraneous. And every single patient that walks through that door has had a miserable childhood. I guarantee it. But usually, the backstory has no bearing on the outcome of the case. The dispo of the patient rests on our predicting the future."

The resident is still looking at me like I am an ogre. I stammer to add more, to make him understand me. "It's ridiculous, really, but that's my job. I need to step back and look at the big picture. I can't get bogged down in the 'oh-the-humanity' response."

"I get it. You've got to hide your love away." He smiles.

"Pretty much, yeah." Maybe he does understand. We do speak the same language, at least.

When I'm in more of a hurry, I care less what my underlings think of me. Tonight would typically be one of those nights, but I want this guy to like me, or at least not to hate me, especially if he's a Beatles fan. I want him to understand that I'm not really heartless. I do care, more than anyone seems to know. I just also care about getting the job done.

"Listen." I search for the right lyric. "I *know* that it's a fool who plays it cool by making his world a little colder. But that's what works for me. This is how I'm choosing to deal with this war zone, y'know? It's the only way I can manage working down here year after year."

He's nodding. We're good. Now I can move along, admitting, discharging, going about my business, walking my tightrope.

When we're even busier, and I don't care how I'm perceived, it goes more like this: "I've got no time for trivialities; I don't want to hear the pitiful backstory. Cut to the chase. Are they suicidal?"

"No."

"Homicidal?"

"No."

"Unable to care for themselves due to psychosis? Presence of severe medical illness exacerbated by psychiatric issues?"

"Nope."

"Then you gotta let 'em go. There's no room at the inn. Tonight is one of those "No Vacancy" nights. If Mary and Joseph end up on triage, they're gonna get T-and-R'd."

Waiting for Laces

By the time the HBO documentary on Bellevue is completed, Lucy is long gone. They dedicate it to her, which I appreciate. She is a central character in the film, just as she was in my life. I miss her terribly, and it is comforting to watch the documentary and see her again, to remember her before she got sick, and bald, and thin and frail.

At the screening, Sheila Nevins of HBO introduces the film. She says something that sticks with me for days afterwards: "There is not much difference between any one of us here today and the patients at Bellevue. We just know enough to put away our imaginary friends if someone knocks on our door."

I admire Sheila, a powerful woman heading up a potent network. Could she be correct in her assessment of what differentiates "us" and "them"? Is it merely that some of us know how to keep our mouths shut? If any of us shared with a psychiatrist every intimate thought we had, our darkest secrets, is it possible we would still be judged safe and sane? There are plenty of times we feel murderous rage, or we think it would be easier if we didn't exist anymore. It's a common fantasy to see ourselves driving the car over the edge of the embankment or into oncoming traffic. Using the criteria of danger to self or others for involuntary commitment, any of these impulses and fantasies is enough to buy you a short stay in the hospital's inpatient psych ward. On the other hand, as long as you keep them to yourself, you can walk around the city freely.

There are many nights at Bellevue when I will listen to a patient strenuously explain to me, "I don't belong here. I'm not crazy. This is all a misunderstanding." Plenty of times, that is indeed the case. Things are said in the heat of the moment, or while drunk or high, that the patient isn't planning to carry out. People are brought to the Bellevue psych ER to be evaluated, and, hopefully, a thorough assessment will reveal the truth.

On one Saturday evening, a man shares a cigarette with a stranger in a bar and ends up dancing naked on top of a car. The cigarette has PCP in it, which luckily shows up in his urine tox screen, helping to explain his behavior. The man has no psychiatric history and I speak to the couple he babysits for to prove it. No matter how psychologically healthy you think you are, circumstances can transpire that will bring you to Bellevue. Hopefully, the doctor in charge will know what to do with you when you get there.

EMS brings in a patient who is on a street corner preaching to passersby about how they should divest themselves of their worldly possessions. He gives away his wallet and watch in the process. When I triage him, I learn that he has eaten several "magic mushrooms" that contain the hallucinogen psilocybin. He has taken them prior to going into a Chelsea art gallery, the Chapel of Sacred Mirrors. The psychedelic artwork within, by Alex Grey, is intense, spiritual, and inspirational, and the combination of the art and the drugs has pulled him onto another plane.

Transformed by the mystical experience, he ends up proselytizing enthusiastically in public. He wants to share with others what he has learned, and that is where he gets himself into trouble. A different psychiatrist might have misdiagnosed him as manic, restraining, medicating, and admitting him, but I have been to the Chapel more than once. I know how moving an experience it can be, never mind the psilocybin. I speak with him gently as his trip slowly ebbs, helping him to navigate his reentry, alighting in a city hospital with no money or identification. He stays in touch with me for months afterwards, grateful that I was there to protect him when he soared beyond the bounds of proscribed public behavior.

There is a diaphanous membrane between sane and insane. It is the flimsiest of barriers, and because any one of us can break through at any given time, it scares all of us. We all lie somewhere on the spectrum,

and our position can shift gradually or suddenly. There is no predicting which of us will be afflicted with dementia or schizophrenia, who
will become incapacitated with depression or panic attacks, or become
suicidal, manic, or addicted. None of these states of mind are uncommon, and all of us have friends and family who are suffering with some
degree of psychiatric illness. Many of us should be grateful for our relative mental health.

The reality is this: All of us, to some degree, are mentally ill. We get
paranoid, anxious, depressed, and insomniac. We alternate between delusions of grandeur and crippling self-doubt, we suffer from paralyzing
fears and embarrassing neuroses. We all have compulsions to do things
we know we shouldn't, and there are millions of us with addictions,
whether to gambling, drinking, dieting, or playing Second Life. Every
one of us has psychiatric symptoms, many of them serious enough to
warrant attention, even if they are not incapacitating. But few of us are
willing to let on that we are suffering. This secrecy and shame com-
pounds our avoidance of those who have been officially diagnosed as
mentally ill. (In family therapy, where the whole family is considered
dysfunctional, there is typically one member considered the "identified
patient," who may have a diagnosis or be taking medication, but everyone else in the family is seen as a participant in the dysfunction, too. As
in family therapy, so too in the world. Some people may be the "identified patients," but we should understand that we are all dysfunctional,
to some extent, individually and collectively.)

We avoid dealing with psychiatric patients because we hate to see
things in others that we don't want to see in ourselves: weakness, need,
despair, aggression. Our experiences with the psychiatrically ill often
fill us with dread; they confront us with our own terror of reaching a
catastrophically altered state from which there is no return. We should
be compassionate to those who stumble out of our lockstep. Yet in our
culture, the mentally ill are demonized and shunned. They are ostracized and marginalized as a by-product of our primal fear of going
crazy ourselves. It is the nightmare of our own "shadow self," as Jung
called it, that allows us to treat others so harshly.

Families who would typically care for their own turn their backs on
children or siblings who have lost their grip on reality. It is too frightening and emotionally draining to tend to their needs. These persistently,
chronically ill patients are then left to fend for themselves, relying on

the shelters, hospitals, and soup kitchens to become their caretakers—their new makeshift families. This is how America does it. The hospitals and outpatient clinics substitute for the parents, who are unable or unwilling to tend to their own psychiatric casualties. And it is painful, first and foremost for the patients. I learned this simple fact in my first year of residency at Mount Sinai. Rounding on our patients in the ward, we asked a man with schizophrenia if anything was hurting him.

"Yes," he replied. "My family doesn't come to see me."

Not all countries treat their disabled in this way. Jeremy and I took our first trip together to Vietnam in 1996. I could see how differently the Asian people dealt with the mentally ill. The "patients" were kept with their families, absorbed within the community, their impact diluted among its healthier members. I would discover them in the villages, where they were assigned menial jobs and managed and attended to by their peers. It is a better system than ours, which lumps all the mentally ill together and concentrates them in state hospitals, nursing homes, and adult homes, where they feed off the insanity of their neighbors.

Instead of integrating them among us, we shutter our psychiatric patients away so that we will not have to be reminded of all that can go wrong with our own minds and brains. It is unfair, not just to those who are in some way mentally "defective," but to us all. I have learned a tremendous amount about myself and the world, about what is important in life and in love, by spending time talking to people with broader worldviews than my own, and that certainly includes the patients I have met at Bellevue. Too quickly, we take away the civil liberties of others due to our collective phobia about insanity, and about altered states in general. This is the basic fear that also fuels our war on drugs, and it is shortsighted and impractical.

We are shortchanging ourselves as a culture by not taking better care of our own psyches, and of the psychiatrically wounded among us. But it's not an easy job, obviously, to fix their wounds. Nearly every shift, I'm asking myself, What do I do with this patient now that he has shown up here in my ER? What does he need from us right now? Unfortunately, the most common answer is: He needs a childhood transplant, he needs to start over—with loving parents this time, in a caring, nurturing environment.

Most psychiatric patients, especially addicts, alcoholics, and criminals, have horrendous histories of neglect and physical and sexual abuse.

Since there's no way to fix that after the fact, it's a lot harder to fix them. Many of the addicts and alcoholics that I triage don't seem all that interested in getting into treatment, or sticking with a program long enough to make real changes in their lives. Letting them sleep in the ER for a night or two rarely works miracles, and one thing I got used to early in the game at Bellevue was seeing some patients over and over: the drunks who'd show up regularly, the crack addicts who'd come in like clockwork when their checks ran out. I learned to regard the revolving door of my workplace with equanimity. I was not going to be able to change a damn thing, more often than not.

"I'm a cog in the machine; I am a spoke in the wheel." I chant my mantra in front of the nurses as I twirl in a circle, waving my arms like Shiva. Between the bureaucracy of working in a huge city hospital and the recidivism of the patients, I develop my own version of the serenity prayer: *Help me learn to accept that I cannot alter the machine, and I will try my hardest to make sure that the machine does not alter me.*

Treated and Released

It is June 27, 2005, my last Monday morning sign-out. July first is next week, but just as I planned last winter, I have not re-upped for another year in Bedlam. I am O.T.D.

I often joked that I'd be working at Bellevue until I was a stooped-over, osteoporotic old woman, and when I said it, I usually believed it, but I've finally worked my last weekend. I've decided to trade in the psychotics for neurotics: I'm going to do full-time private practice. I always assumed I'd stay hospital-based, mired in academia, teaching and performing clinical research, but my path is pulling me in a different direction. I feel as though I'm heading out to pasture, and I'm not even forty.

I tell people that the reason I am leaving is because of Molly; I need to alter my schedule to accommodate hers. She'll be starting kindergarten in the fall, and we have decided that we'd prefer her to go to school in New York City, which means reversing our schedule and spending our weekdays in the city and our weekends upstate. That in turn means I can't keep working my weekend shifts at Bellevue, but working weekdays at Bellevue doesn't make any sense financially. I can work in my private practice three days a week and still spend plenty of time with my family. And I'm starting to feel that I can be a better doctor in my office than I can in the ER, with a chance of effecting real and lasting change in people's lives.

I'm looking forward to luxuriating in long-term care instead of triage. I see now that I need the follow-up. I need my people to get better and stay better. I've done enough triaging and crisis intervention to last a lifetime, and I'm done passing the patient along to another doctor once I've arrived at a diagnosis. I want to do the whole job now. In my private practice, once I settle on the right medication to manage symptoms, there are still years of sessions, getting to understand the patient's situation, unique stresses, struggles with weight, libido, and balancing work and family. Their prescription regimen is often tailored to help weather particular storms, and I want to be with them, helping them to navigate through the choppy waters, instead of fishing them out of the stormy sea, letting them sleep on the deck, and then dropping them off at the marina to await another boat.

These past few months, knowing I would be leaving CPEP soon, I was constantly on the lookout for reminders about why I was going. Like waiting until after the holidays to break up with a boyfriend, once I knew I was going to end it, it got harder to stick around and easier to rationalize my impending departure. There are countless things I've put up with year after year that I won't miss: more prisoners, more paperwork, more complicated computer maneuvers. They've been snowballing over time, getting worse, conveniently, in the few months leading up to my planned escape.

But here's the thing that is tipping the scales the most: I've transformed significantly, and I'm afraid permanently. It's not you, Bellevue, it's me; *I've* changed. The combination of motherhood and psychotherapy has brought down a one-two punch that is making me incompatible with emergency psychiatric work. My hormone-fueled maternal instinct blossomed during my stay at the hospital, and I now can't shrug things off the way I used to.

When I started my job at CPEP, I made a conscious decision to alter my exterior. I inured myself to the tragedy that walked through the doors. That hard-ass persona allowed me to go about my business weekend after weekend. But my three years of psychotherapy with Mary allowed me to see this act for what it was—a defense. And she taught me, through each of my undignified transgressions, that acting this way does not help my patients.

Oscar Wilde says, "Experience is the name everyone gives to their mistakes." With every mistake, we must surely be learning, right? Maybe I took longer than others, but eventually I did grow from my experiences, and over time, I softened up my rough edges. But those years of therapy left me with some tender patches that were painfully unprotected. My suit of armor didn't seem to fit like it did before.

And then motherhood came along, further dilating those soft spots. Something about the physical act of giving birth and nurturing two infants had turbocharged my capacity for empathy. My carefully constructed cynicism and distance started to crack. By 2005, I was simply not the same person I was in 1996. I went from being the prison warden to being the den mother. After two pregnancies and four years of nursing, it was a lot harder to pretend I was one of the guys; being butch just didn't fly anymore. I couldn't strut around like I used to, keys jangling, invincible. I had adopted a more caring and approachable bedside manner in my private practice, and I couldn't shift gears gracefully between my two offices, even if I did have two different bags to take there, accessories to my two different personas.

And then, of course, there was September 11. I remember soon after, sitting in a bathtub with Molly. I pictured a huge jet engine roaring through our high-rise apartment building. I could imagine the cockpit crashing into our bathroom, killing us instantly, or worse, killing only her, and it took my breath away. I sat in that tub, clutching her to my chest, breathless and panicked. I could not bear to lose her.

Motherhood taught me about love, and 9/11 taught me about loss. The terrorists showed us all how quickly life could be taken, and how much it could hurt. After that Tuesday, it seemed, I could no longer look at the lives ruined at Bellevue with my usual casual glance. Every one of those patients had a family somewhere, and a mother, which made it exponentially harder to dampen my heartstrings. I couldn't deliver my news over the telephone to the concerned parents with the same degree of remove, the clinician's professional level of indifference. Because I was now a parent too, I couldn't detach like I needed to. I would hang up from a phone call completely drained, full of sorrow for what they'd have to go through in the years to come.

I hated coming home to my kids emotionally wrung out, trying to blot out the memories of the patients I had treated. We'd be at the playground and my kids would be in the sandbox, but I'd be in the hospital—I couldn't stop reliving what I had seen or done at work. I was having too much bleed-through between my work and home life, regardless of how organized my closet was. No matter which backpack

I was carrying, insanity intruded into my life, as it impinges on us all, like it or not.

I have to admit, I never quite found that middle ground between hard and hypersensitive. I know there is a compassionate place well beyond sadism, an expanse of territory way past empathic failure and just short of giving till it hurts, but for the life of me, I can't find that place when I am at CPEP. Despite Mary's best efforts, it has remained elusive. I have to simply accept that I can't manage caring for the patients, for myself, and for my family the way I need to.

It's time to let someone else take over.

And so, using my family as an excuse, I make my gracious exit.

I try to make my last sign-out memorable, pulling out all the stops, squeezing in jokes wherever I can. When I'm done, there's an awkward silence. One of the attendings, a woman of course, clears her throat to say a few words.

"As you all know, it's Doctor Holland's last day today. She's been here nine years."

"Longer than any other CPEP attending," I chime in. It is an accomplishment I am proud of, and I have joked with the head nurse for months about wanting a plaque to prove it.

"Well, we want to wish you well, of course," she says, "and also, I feel like someone should say something about Lucy. You're the last doctor here who actually worked with her, and you were her good friend. You're our last tie to Lucy, and with you going, it really is the end of an era."

I did not expect this. No one warned me there would be Lucy talk. I immediately get misty-eyed, which is the last thing I want right now. I want to leave with my head held high, strong, dignified. I swallow hard and think about something, anything, other than my dead friend.

"We'll really miss your Monday morning sign-outs. It's not going to be the same around here without you."

"I'm counting on it," I choke out.

I leave the nurses' station and head for the locker room where there are bagels and coffee to celebrate my last day. There are many hugs, and some good stories about my greatest hits, but there is no plaque.

Castles Made of Sand

We arrive at Cape Cod ahead of the Fourth of July traffic—not that I could see any of the cars behind me. Our station wagon is loaded to the brim with clothes, sand toys, and bicycles; the windsurfer is attached to the roof by a tangle of bungee cords.

We've been telling Jojo about the beach for days, and even though he is only fifteen months old, he seems to remember this place, somehow. He makes the sign for water as we get out of the car.

The four of us walk around the house to the porch and say hello to the ocean. There is a strong breeze, and there are plenty of sailboats on the bay.

"How about if you set up the windsurfer and I'll make up the beds?" I offer to Jeremy.

Molly entertains Jojo on the lawn while Jeremy and I unpack the car and start to set up house.

It is early evening by the time the kids are fed, the bags are unpacked, and the beds are made. Jojo is taking a nap, and Molly and Jeremy are changing into their swimsuits. It is time for me to do the thing that I love most at the Cape.

I lug the board down to the beach and attach the sail. My water shoes and gloves, from the shelf above the washing machine in the garage, just where I left them last Labor Day, are dry and crackly, caked with salt and sand, but they soften immediately as I dunk my hands and feet in the shallow water. I nervously scan the ocean floor for critters as I walk the sailboard out into the deeper water. With my back to the wind, I climb onto the board and stand there for a minute, savoring the moment before the sail is pulled up. I can see the house with its wraparound porch, the beach peppered with children digging in the sand. All around me is air and water, sea and sky.

I remember to breathe.

I squat down to untangle the rope, composing a sea chantey as I prepare to pull up the sail, imagining pirates on a ship singing, "What shall we do with the drunken sailor?" as they hoist the main. Hand over hand I pull on the rope, my weight back, guiding the mast from horizontal to vertical, until I swap the rope for mast and boom. I reposition my feet as I slowly pull the boom toward me, catching the breeze in the sail.

Steering the board with my feet, tilting the mast to assist in the navigation, I snake the windsurfer between the boats still moored in the bay.

As the bay opens up onto the ocean, there are no more sailboats and motorboats to squeeze by. My obstacles are all behind me. It is just the open sea, the breeze, and I.

I tilt my head so my hair blows away from my face. The wind is misty, salty. I inhale the brine deep into my lungs, thinking how the Bellevue AES docs would administer saline intravenously as the first order of business. There is salt in our blood, in our sweat, and in our tears. Even when we are babies inside the womb, we are cushioned in an oceanic haven.

Here, riding on top of the water, harnessing the breeze, the zephyrs stroking my hair, I have found my asylum, my shelter. Whether on a broad reach or a close haul, as long as I stay out at sea, I am alee, safe from the storm. I will not be rained on by debris from explosions; I will not be required to clean up the psychic fallout from the traumas. I have left the land of four-point restraints and medications, of poverty and despair. I am responsible for no one, for none of it. I have no decisions to make that will alter the course of anyone's life, only the course of my small craft, upwind or down.

I have signed out my private practice for the month of July. My patient load is zero. I have closed one chapter of my life, but I have not yet opened the next. I suppose this is the whole idea of summer vacation: not working. I can focus on caring for myself and for my family. I can get some perspective now that I am away from the hospital. Determining who is sane, who is ill, who needs to be locked up for their own good, and who may run free, like the wind . . . this is no longer my bailiwick. Now I decide what to make for dinner, and whether to do laundry today or tomorrow.

Oh, God, will I die of boredom? Sky of blue and sea of green, every one of us has all we need. But will it be enough for me?

The sun hangs fat and low on the horizon as the Technicolor display begins. Wisps of clouds decorate the sky, layered with hints of the vermillion, fuchsia, and tangerine to come. I search for the moon as my board bounces on the rolling waves, carrying me out to sea, farther away.

Actually, too far away.

I have been sailing west for too long. I need to reach the shore before it gets too dark to see and be seen, just as I needed to leave Bellevue before I faded into the background, before we became the same drab color.

I head into the wind and come about clumsily. It'll take a few days to work the kinks out of my form, but at least I haven't fallen in yet. My T-shirt is dry as I approach the shore, my forearms aching.

I look behind me once more, to take in the mango-papaya sunset. It is the medical new year, Independence Day weekend, and I am not going back to the hospital. I'm not a cog in the machine anymore, but I still feel my wheels spinning. I remind myself: It will take some time to work those kinks out too. Head for shore, and everything will fall into place.

Jeremy and Molly are frolicking like dolphins in the waves as I glide past them, hooting and crowing.

"Yay, Mommy!" Molly shouts.

I grin triumphantly as I release the sail, pushing it away from me as I fall backwards into the water.

Paperback Writer

It's a snowy Sunday afternoon in January, and I haven't stepped foot in Bellevue for six months.

My life has slid into a predictable routine. I see patients mid week, take the kids up to the house on Friday, and come back Sunday night to do it again. Monday is my errand day; we have a sitter to watch Jojo, and I've started back up with Pilates. My life is simpler, and it feels infinitely safer, but I'm not sure it's better. And there's no going back. I will never have a job like CPEP again. Not only do I miss my Bellevue comrades, I miss the rush of being in charge, talking to the cops, feeling decisive, helping the people the rest of the city has avoided and discarded. I miss never knowing what's going to happen next.

Like a junkie in withdrawal, I find it easy to glorify the good old days spent high on adrenaline with my crew. It will take some more time to adjust to my new life.

CPEP was all about diagnosis not treatment, triaging not fixing. Most of my job was simply determining who's in and who's out. My life isn't like that anymore; it's not so black-and-white. Now, it's all about the long view: raising a family, writing books, following my private practice patients month after month. I'm treating people who are no longer lost to follow-up. I am responsible for the outcome, good or bad. Luckily, my patients are getting better and staying well, for the most part. They are grateful to me for my ministrations, and their families are likely relieved that I'm helping to shoulder the burden of maintaining their mental health.

Still, I know someone else could be doing this type of work, someone more sedate. Not everyone is built for Bellevue like I was. Should I have stayed because I could? Am I really contributing in the same way now? I still find myself talking to the homeless schizophrenics on the street, telling them to head to Bellevue when they look like they're going south. They're my people, and I can't help but do a little community outreach while I'm waiting for the subway.

It's snowing like crazy here at the house, and I'm supposed to give a Monday morning lecture to the residents at CPEP, something I've agreed to do in order to keep up my voluntary faculty position. More important, I am meeting Nancy for breakfast at the coffee shop before I teach, at the end of her Sunday overnight shift. Though I'm dying to catch up with her, it will have to wait. Jeremy and I are pretending we're snowed-in so our whole family can play hooky from school and work. I'll find another Monday morning to head down to the hospital.

I call Nancy to reschedule. An unfamiliar voice answers the phone, "CPEP." A new clerk.

"Hi. This is Doctor Holland; I used to work there. You may not know me." It's the first time I've had to speak like this to someone at CPEP, and it feels awful. "Is Nancy working tonight, do you know?"

I am put on hold. The new clerk is afraid to give out any information about a CPEP employee, because she has no idea who's calling. I appreciate her reluctance, actually. I'd want the same level of security if someone were trying to track me down, asking if I'd be there tonight.

I'm on hold for a good long time, listening to the Bellevue propaganda that plays ad nauseam, in Spanish, Mandarin, and English. When I was working there and had to put someone on hold, I used to just put the phone down on the counter, instead of pressing the hold button, as long as I was feeling merciful; that recorded message can seem like torture after you've heard it a dozen times.

A man gets on the phone and says, "Hello, Miss? Yeah, so, um . . . no one here has any idea who Doctor Holland is. We have no record of any Doctor Holland working here."

I am speechless.

"You're kidding me," I whine. "No one there knows who I am?" It is a narcissist's worst nightmare. My so-called legacy is already nonexistent, faded into oblivion a mere six months after I leave. It simply cannot be.

"Wait a minute! Who is this?" I demand.

"It's Henry," my friend says, and I can hear his smile. I've known Henry for thirteen years; he was my chief resident during my second year of training at Mount Sinai. Actually, I'm the one who recommended he get a job moonlighting at CPEP. "In fact, I'm looking at your picture right now," he says. He is holding a copy of my Ecstasy book in his hands, which he has taken from the bookshelf in the nurses' station.

"What's going on there today?" I ask hungrily.

"Oh, the usual," he deadpans. "We had a stabbing."

"Weapon?" I ask, sliding into CPEP shorthand-speak.

"Pen. Hidden between the guy's gluteus maximi."

I like his pluralization of "maximus." Nice touch. "How'd he get that?"

"We figure it came out of the social work office. It was unlocked."

"We're going to have to step up security," I say, as if I still work there and need to send out a memo: *Guard your pens. They can be used to stab patients in the neck.*

The patient who did the stabbing is the same man who was arrested for running into the UN naked. I'd heard about him in the news and assumed he was brought to Bellevue, but I'm surprised that he has become violent, and mention this to Henry. "Usually the naked guys are harmless."

"Yeah, you figure anyone who's willing to be so vulnerable wouldn't be very paranoid."

I realize we are on the same page. It is bittersweet, to be immediately understood, yet distanced.

"I miss it there." I sigh. I remember the buzz of the hive, the acuteness of the patients, the predictable level of chaos, punctuated by the unpredictable. I think about Chuck, the last night we worked together, turning away to hide his tears as I left the nurses' station to turn in for the night. "Every Saturday at six, I still feel the pull of the hospital. I feel like I'm supposed to get in my car and go to Bellevue so I can see everyone."

"Well, we all miss you, too, you know," Henry says.

"And you really had me going with that 'No one here knows who Doctor Holland is.' I couldn't believe there was already no one there who remembered me."

"Oh, I don't think anyone here will be forgetting you anytime soon," Henry assures me.

"You better not," I threaten faux-menacingly, hanging up the phone.

I will never forget Bellevue. And I couldn't bear the asymmetry if my passage through the hospital had no impact, my footprints already washed away by the changing tides of each successive shift. I don't want CPEP to forget me, and I surely don't want them to forget Lucy. If I close my eyes, I can see her pulling down the New Testament from the nurses' station bookshelf, randomly opening up a page to guide her. I want *Weekends at Bellevue* to sit alongside it on that shelf, a testament to our time spent together at the hospital.

My nine years at CPEP, like an extended gestation, helped to make me what I am—a better doctor, a better mother, and a writer. I walked into that asylum one person, and I walked out another. I didn't alter the machine—I'm not sure anyone could have—but it surely had its way with me.

Glossary

2 PC—two physician certificate. An involuntary admission lasting up to sixty days.

5 and 2—5 milligrams of the antipsychotic Haldol and 2 milligrams of the antianxiety sedative Ativan.

9.13—voluntary admission.

9.39—involuntary admission, lasting up to two weeks.

9.40—seventy-two-hour Hold. An admission to the EOU (extended observation unit).

18 South—an acute ward with Asian-language-speaking staff. Mandarin- and Cantonese-speaking patients are preferentially sent here.

19 West—the male forensic unit.

20 East—the dual diagnosis unit (also called the MICA unit, for Mentally Ill, Chemically Abusing patients).

AES—Adult Emergency Services. The medical ER at Bellevue.

Akathisia—an inability to remain still, an uncomfortable physical compulsion to pace, or shake one's legs arising as a side effect from antipsychotic and some antidepressant medications.

AOB—Alcohol on Breath.

Attending—a doctor who has finished residency, often the doctor in charge.

Blue room—Department of Corrections holding area.

Bridge up—a person on a bridge about to jump.

Bundle—ten bags of heroin.

Camisole—a euphemism for straightjacket.

CPEP—Comprehensive Psychiatric Emergency Program. The psychiatric ER at Bellevue.

Debridement—removing infected or dead tissue from a wound.

D.O.C.—Department of Corrections. NYC prison guards, who work at Rikers and Bellevue.

DNR—Do Not Resuscitate. An order on a medical chart instructing doctors and nurses to forgo heroic measures if the patient is dying.

EDP—emotionally disturbed person, NYPD terminology for a psychiatric patient.

Eloping—a euphemism for escaping a locked ward.

EMS—Emergency Medical Services. NYC ambulances and their drivers, who are often EMTs (emergency medical technicians).

EOU—Extended Observation Unit. CPEP's six-bedded unit for seventy-two-hour holds.

ESU—Emergency Services Unit. When NYPD needs backup, they call ESU, which helps to subdue and restrain patients.

Hold—an involuntary status to observe the patient for up to twenty-four hours.

MR—mentally retarded.

MTA—Metropolitan Transportation Authority. NYC bus, subway, and train system.

Malinger—to fake being ill, or mentally ill.

Malingerer—someone who fakes illness for personal gain.

Moonlighter—a doctor who is hired to work extra shifts during nights, weekends, and holidays. This can be a resident or an attending.

NYFD—New York Fire Department.

Neuropathic—a symptom coming from nerve irritation or damage, a neuropathy.

O.T.D.—Out the Door, discharged.

PINS—Person in Need of Service. A parent petitions the court to step in to help with child supervision.

Prn's—as-needed medications, as opposed to standing medications, often given for agitation, anxiety, or alcohol withdrawal symptoms.

Psych techs—the staff in the nondetainable area who have the most patient contact.

Resident—a doctor who is still in training, but has chosen a specialty (e.g., a surgical resident, a psychiatric resident). Residencies typically last three or four years.

Shark—sociopath. Often a malingerer. Sociopaths are not truly mentally ill, but their lives are disorganized and they may prey on the patients.

Snake pit—an old-fashioned way of referring to an asylum or mental hospital.

Standing medications—those medications given daily, as opposed to prn medications.

Acknowledgments

First of all, I want to thank every single patient I have ever come into contact with, bar none. You enriched me, and I am forever in your debt. If I have helped you get back on your intended path, I am pleased. If I thwarted you, frustrated you, or much worse, I am deeply sorry. I hope it helps you to know that I am still struggling to become a better, kinder, gentler person now than I was then.

My agent and friend, Kirsten Manges, did her job and then some, helping me to land a book deal and making my dreams come true, basically. At Bantam, Beth Rashbaum, editor summa cum laude, saw the potential in the manuscript that came her way, and helped me to make it shine. Michael Cunningham helped to champion this book and served as ambassador to the publishing world.

Thanks to my readers and advisors: Jessica Wolff, an astute line editor and advisor who helped me early in the process, and Kate O'Connell, who gave me great advice about narrative arcs and character development. Simone Solondz boldly recommended I cut out some of the more provocative and objectionable stories, Marjorie Ingall provided an equally brave critique, Elizabeth Stein helped me to make some painful cuts and sutures, and Jen Dohne and Collective Copies of Amherst assisted with manuscript preparation.

Richard Gehr and Gary Greenberg helped me to shape and mold this book. William Ridinger proffered tireless, meticulous notes for multiple rounds of rewrites, and is a heckuva pen pal. Steven Fressola, Joel Bassuk, and Michael Hogan were a great cheering section. David Rhoads, Jim Fadiman, and John Howell provided much-needed eleventh-hour critiques and support.

There were certain psychiatrists throughout my training who were particularly inspirational: Ed Schweizer at Penn, John Benson at Temple, and Jack Hirschowitz and Ann Callahan at Mount Sinai.

To my husband, Jeremy, thank you for all your sage advice and balance.

To my parents, sisters, and my children, Molly and Joe, I am blessed to have your love and understanding.

About the Author

JULIE HOLLAND, M.D., is a psychiatrist specializing in psychopharmacology. An assistant professor of psychiatry at New York University School of Medicine, she spent her weekends running the psychiatric emergency room at Bellevue Hospital for nine years. She is the editor of *Ecstasy: The Complete Guide, A Comprehensive Look at the Risks and Benefits of MDMA*. She lectures widely and has been quoted in *Time, Harper's, Los Angeles Times,* and *The Wall Street Journal*. Holland has appeared as a medical expert on the *Today* show, *Good Morning America,* and CNN. She is in a private practice in New York City and lives with her husband and two children in the Hudson Valley.